Y0-BFJ-023

As Taught
in Siddha Meditation
Ashrams

Published by SYDA Foundation ▪ South Fallsburg, New York

© 1981 SYDA Foundation
All rights reserved
Third printing 1985; revised edition
Compiled by Prema Mandrell and Sarala Troy
Illustrations by Julie Hagan
Cover design by Asesha Conroy

Published by SYDA Foundation
P.O. Box 600, South Fallsburg, NY 12779
ISBN: 0914602-72-1 /LCCN: 81-51182

About Swami Muktananda

Swami Muktananda began his search for God at an early age. When he was only fifteen, his yearning was so strong that he set out in search of a Guru. To strengthen his commitment, he took the vows of monkhood at the ashram of Siddharudha Swami in Hubli. Over the course of the next twenty-five years he traveled all over India, meeting many spiritual teachers and saints. He studied Vedanta and the other systems of Indian philosophy, yoga, Ayurvedic medicine, as well as mundane sciences such as horticulture, music, and the martial arts. Although he mastered many forms of knowledge, and met many great men, it wasn't until he met his Guru that he found a being who embodied the knowledge he was looking for. That being was Bhagawan Nityananda of Ganeshpuri. After spending some time in Bhagawan Nityananda's company, he received *shaktipat* from him; with that initiation, his real spiritual practices began. Over the next nine years, Swami Muktananda had incredible inner experiences which culminated in his attainment of God-realization. Shortly thereafter, Bhagawan Nityananda gave him a small piece of land with three rooms close to Ganeshpuri, which became Gurudev Siddha Peeth. Before Bhagawan Nityananda took *mahasamadhi* (died) in 1961, he passed the power of the Siddha lineage on to Swami Muktananda.

Swami Muktananda toured the world three times, teaching Siddha meditation and awakening people's divine inner energy through *shaktipat* initiation. In May 1982, a few months before Baba Muktananda himself took *mahasamadhi,* he passed the power of the Siddha lineage to Swami Chidvilasananda and Swami Nityananda. Swami Nityananda retired in 1985. Now Swami Chidvilasananda, or Gurumayi as she is affectionately called, continues the work — giving people the experience of their own unlimited inner depths through meditation and *shaktipat.* Wherever Gurumayi goes, people receive that grace, that unconditional love, that experience of their own divinity which is the hallmark of the Siddha tradition.

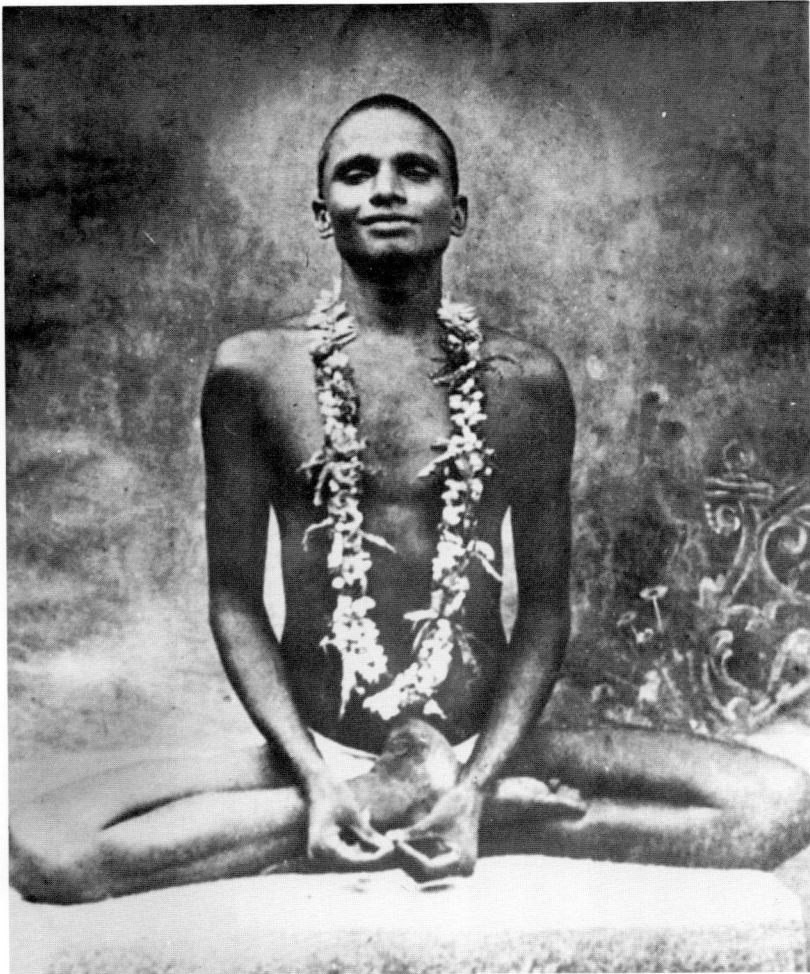

Swami Muktananda's Guru, Bhagawan Nityananda, in *Siddhasana*.

In the *Bhagavad Gita*, Lord Krishna compares the body to a field. He says, "O Arjuna, this body is called 'the field.' " This statement is worth thinking about seriously and carefully. Why does He call the body "the field"?

First, think about a field of earth. It is always ready to cooperate with us. It has no desires or demands of its own. It never prevents you from doing whatever you like with it. You can turn the field into an apple orchard or a flower garden. You can subdivide it into residential plots, and people will come and live there. You can build an ashram on it, and many people will come and do spiritual practices. Or you can make a cemetery, and it will receive the dead. If you do not do anything, the field will become overgrown with bushes and thorns. Whatever you give to the field will be given back to you.

So Krishna called the body "the field." Just like that piece of ground, the body is also a field which always cooperates with us. A man can train it and become a wrestler in this body. He can become an artist, a singer, a wise man, or a priest in this body. He can become a good man or a bad man. He can remember God and even become God. This is the body which God has given us; we can do whatever we like with it. Think about it. What is there that a human being has not done in the body?

So take good care of this field. An ancient sage once said, "The body is the primary means to enlightenment." There is magnificent divinity in it, which is called "the knower of the field," and we should set out to find that truth, the ultimate reality, God. If we meditate, if we sow meditation in this field, we can see and attain that great divinity.

— Swami Muktananda

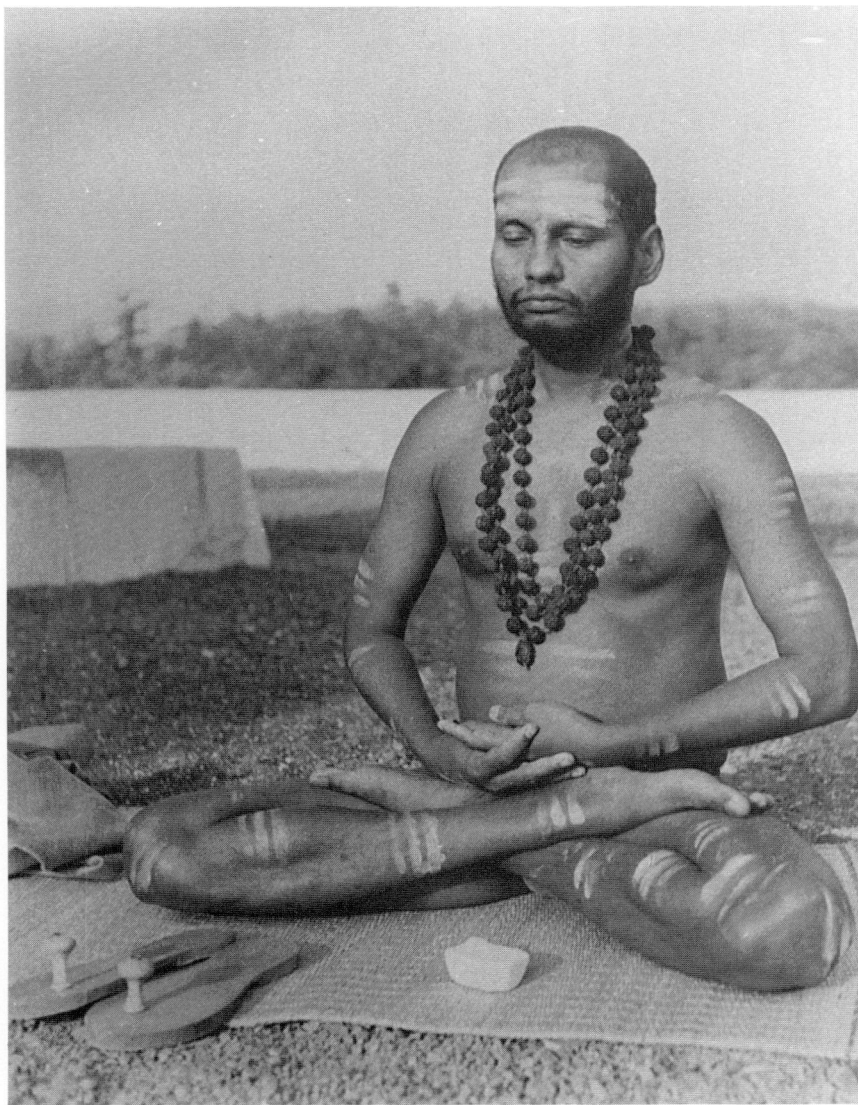

Swami Muktananda in *Padmasana*,
Ganeshpuri, 1956.

Contents

Preface   viii
Introduction   1
Practical Advice   3

Surya Namaskar   4

Postures   11
Warming-Up   12
Standing Postures   16
Sitting Postures   28
Forward Bending Postures   33
Backward Bending Postures   40
Spinal Twist Postures   44
Shoulderstand Series   48
Reclining Postures   54

**Relaxation and Breathing
Exercises**   59
The Corpse Pose   60
Full Yogic Breath   61
Bhastrika   63

Meditation Postures   65

Siddha Meditation   71

**Questions and Answers with
Swami Muktananda**   75

Appendix A
Suggested Routine   81
Appendix B
Surya Namaskar Series   82
Index   84
SYDA Publications   86
Major Ashrams   87

Preface

Hatha Yoga is much more than physical exercise. Its effects on the mind and body are surprisingly deep and varied. Simply put, it changes people from the inside out. Faces become brighter; hearts open; minds become still; agressive people become calmer; lazy, tired people experience a freshness and strength; and, with continued practice, overall "dis-ease" and discomfort gradually disappear. Students who previously accepted aches and pains as normal discover a new sense of physical and mental well-being.

The goal of all yogas, including Hatha Yoga, is to bring us to a state of union with our own essential nature—the inner Self. Practices such as meditation, contemplation and self-inquiry lead toward that state by making the mind still, allowing the Self to be revealed. In Hatha Yoga, the technique of self-inquiry, for example, can be applied to both "outer" and "inner" postures. Observing the outer posture, we ask: Am I standing straight? Is my weight balanced? Are my shoulders relaxed? Am I experiencing tension in any part of my body?

Having made the physical adjustments, our focus turns to the subtle inner posture, the posture of the mind: Is my mind one-pointed? Am I chasing after thoughts? What is the nature of the thoughts arising? Am I able to witness them? Continuous self-inquiry allows the body and mind to be drawn into balance. Practiced in this way, Hatha Yoga is truly a meditation in action.

Such practices alone, however, only rarely bring full enlightenment. The key to this state, according to nearly all yogic scriptures, is the grace of a perfected Master—a Siddha, one who has reached perfection and can reveal the inherent perfection in others. Contact with such a Siddha master leads to the awakening of the spiritual power, Kundalini, lying dormant within everyone. With this awakening, through a subtle transmission of energy called *shaktipat*, a process of inner unfolding begins, naturally and spontaneously leading us to a state of unity with our innermost nature. Focused attention on physical movement and posture, as presented in this book, helps still the mind. Swami Chidvilasananda says, ". . . Yoga is not better muscles; yoga is a better mind. A better mind is a quiet mind from which everything springs."

This completely revised edition, which contains many new postures, is designed to lead the student gradually from the easy to the more difficult postures. Beginners, older practitioners and those people with weak backs will benefit from using the variations of the poses and props, such as folded blankets and cotton straps. A list of cautions is especially useful for pregnant women or those with physical limitations. Special attention is given to the development of a flexible and straight spine.

This manual presents the way Hatha Yoga is taught in Siddha Meditation Ashrams throughout the world. It is not intended to replace personal instruction but rather to be used for individual practice in conjunction with classes.

—Prema Mandrell

There is a saying in the yoga scriptures: "If the body is weak, if the veins and nerves are weak, if there is no strength in the *prana*, the life force, to flow in and out, then how can you derive any joy from living?"

Regardless of what else you may have in your life — wealth, status, endless degrees — if your body isn't healthy, how can you enjoy any of it? Consequently, it is of primary importance for you to keep the body healthy and strong. Some people try to do this through sports, while others practice Hatha Yoga. The *asanas*, or postures, of Hatha Yoga do help to make the body very pure, strong and well-built. Learning the postures also helps you to maintain a good sitting position for meditation and to lead a life of discipline and self-control. At one time I practiced all of the 84 main asanas of Hatha Yoga and, as a result, even now every muscle in my body is under my control.

I find that in America when people talk about Hatha Yoga, they are referring only to the practice of asanas. There is much more to Hatha Yoga than just a few postures. According to the scriptures of Hatha Yoga, the *Hatha Yoga Pradipika* and the *Gheranda Samhita*, even before learning to do the asanas you must first do the six *shatkarmas*, or internal purificatory processes, which are meant to purify, cleanse and balance the humors of the body.

Then, sitting in a proper asana, you must apply the three *bandhas*, or locks, in order to control the flow of *prana*, along with *kumbhaka*, or breath retention. These are the essential techniques of Hatha Yoga. However, there are very few reliable teachers who can teach you these techniques; even if you succeed in finding a good teacher, you have to have a very healthy and strong body in order to practice them. Then even if you exert yourself for many years, there is no guarantee of success.

The goal of Hatha Yoga is the uniting of *ha* and *tha*, which correspond to the right and left nostrils, and the two *nadis* or subtle nerve channels, called *ida* and *pingala*. When these two currents come together, the central nerve, called the *sushumna*, is activated and then the real yoga begins. At that point an inner awakening occurs, and the dormant spiritual energy, Kundalini, begins to unfold. When this happens, you will experience internal yoga; spontaneous purificatory processes will begin to occur and you will experience divine meditation.

Hatha yogis try to bring about this awakening through the various techniques of *bandhas*, *pranayama* and *mudras*, which require great effort, are difficult and can even be dangerous. The scriptures also describe other means, such as repetition of a mantra with great love or intense devotion to God. But the easiest and best method is through *shaktipat* initiation from a Siddha Guru. Through this initiation the Guru transmits his own divine power into the disciple and the inner Kundalini is automatically activated and set into operation.

Just as a seed contains a whole tree in potential form, Kundalini contains all the different forms of yoga, and when She is awakened through the grace of a Guru, She makes all yogas take place spontaneously within you. The process which begins when you receive *shaktipat* is called Siddha Yoga, the perfect yoga. This yoga bears fruit immediately. Siddha Yoga is also called Maha Yoga (great yoga) because it encompasses all other yogas. There are many kinds of yogas: Hatha Yoga, the practice of physical postures; Bhakti Yoga, the path of love; Raja Yoga, which is attained through meditation; Mantra Yoga, Laya Yoga, Jnana Yoga and many others. When the Kundalini is awakened, knowledge of these different yogas comes to you automatically, from the inside.

For example, after *shaktipat* initiation, one may automatically begin to perform various Hatha Yoga asanas, *mudras*, *bandhas* and different kinds of *pranayama*, breath control exercises. These spontaneous movements inspired by the Kundalini are called *kriyas*, and they occur in order to purify and strengthen the body. If you try to practice these techniques on your own on the basis of your limited understanding, you won't really know which ones are good for you. And these techniques are so powerful that they should not even be attempted without the guidance of an adept teacher and strict adherence to the discipline involved. But when these processes occur spontaneously in meditation, through the inspiration of the awakened Kundalini, you automatically perform only those practices which are necessary and appropriate for you. For example, *Sarvangasana* may be the posture which is best suited for my constitution, but I may be practicing *Shirshasana* instead, which is not good for me at all.

In the same way, when the Kundalini becomes active, you may hear the repetition of different mantras inside, which is an experience of Mantra Yoga, or your mind may become absorbed in visions of lights or inner sounds, which are the experiences of Laya Yoga. For a student of Siddha Yoga, these genuine yogic experiences come effortlessly through the grace of the Guru and the Kundalini.

Students often ask me if it is all right for them to practice Hatha Yoga postures, or if they should wait for them to occur spontaneously in meditation. If asana, *bandhas* or *mudras* take place in your meditation, then let them happen. They will purify your body and enable you to hold the Shakti. But if you want to practice some asanas and *Bhastrika* independently, they will be very beneficial in helping to purify and strengthen the physical body and will help you to achieve a steady posture, which is essential for the higher states of meditation. The nerves also become purified, thus ensuring a smooth flow of *prana* throughout the whole body, preparing it for the awakening of Kundalini. Then supreme peace begins to rise up from within, and you will not need to make an effort to meditate; meditation will occur spontaneously.

— Swami Muktananda

Practical Advice

1. For maximum benefit and progress in your Hatha Yoga practice establish a regular routine, preferably at the same time each day.

2. It is best to practice the postures when you arise.

3. Wear loose, comfortable clothing that will allow freedom of movement. Standing poses especially should be practiced barefoot to improve the balance.

4. Practice with an empty stomach if possible; otherwise, advisable intervals are two hours after a light meal, or three to four hours after a full meal.

5. Upon completion of asanas, wait one half hour before eating; after intense *Bhastrika*, wait one full hour before eating.

6. Women should not do strenuous postures, inversions or *Bhastrika* during the first three days of menstruation.

7. Do not practice postures if you have a severe cold, flu or fever, because this is a sign that your body needs rest.

8. Some bodily discomfort may be felt during the intitial stages of practice, such as the stretching of tight hamstrings. However, it is important to distinguish between a health-giving stretch and a sharp, injurious pain. Do not continue to practice a posture when you experience pain in the knees, lower back or neck.

9. Remember to breathe normally throughout the postures — holding the breath creates tension and fatigue.

10. Do not use strain or force at any time, but work within your individual limits. When holding a posture, release into it gradually with each exhalation. If you surrender your will and remain focused on your inner Self, the pose will deepen naturally.

Salutations to the Sun

SURYA NAMASKAR

(*surya*, sun; *namaskar*, salutation — salutations to the sun)

This is a graceful series of movements that people traditionally performed in the early morning, facing the rising sun, as a form of worship. Today, it remains an extremely effective way to activate and loosen every part of the body and to develop breathing capacity. It helps to prepare one for the practice of more difficult and complicated asanas by making the spine flexible and strong. The various movements stimulate the entire body, including all of the systems (endocrine, circulatory, respiratory, digestive, etc.), and greatly assist in loosening the joints and stretching the muscles of the legs. The synchronization of the movements and the rhythm of the breath develops coordination and breath control.

Initially, the various movements should be performed slowly and carefully, and each individual posture perfected. Then the breath can be combined with the movements; always inhale when the chest is expanded and exhale when bending forward. Once the sequence comes easily, allow your own breathing rhythm to guide the speed with which you practice the movements.

Upon arising in the morning, you can execute *Surya Namaskar* rapidly to energize and stimulate the body and mind. In his Ganeshpuri Ashram, Swami Muktananda taught it to the young boys, and encouraged them to practice it rapidly, without sacrificing the precision of each movement. Many of his students perform *Surya Namaskar* 100 times (50 rounds) each morning before meditation. This takes about 20 minutes and has an aerobic effect on the cardiovascular system, similar to that of running. At other times of the day, it can be performed slowly and gracefully to release tension in the muscles and remove fatigue.

A long *Surya Namaskar* should be followed by *Shavasana* for a few minutes, allowing the heartbeat and respiration to gradually return to normal, and relaxing the body completely.

Position 1

- stand with feet parallel, and slightly apart
- place palms together at chest in *namaskar* (prayer) position
- inhale, firm thighs and lift spine
- exhale slowly

Position 2

- inhale, raise arms above head
- keep kneecaps lifted and buttocks firm
- stretch arms up from armpits, and open upper chest

Do not push the pelvis forward, as this might strain the lower back. Keep the pelvis directly over the feet, and concentrate on opening the upper back.

Position 3

- inhale, firm thighs and lift spine
- exhale, bend from hip joints, with arms reaching forward as far as possible
- if hands touch floor easily, place hands beside feet
- keep knees straight and legs fully extended
- let head hang freely, and release into forward bend position

Avoid bending from the waist, which creates tremendous pressure on the spinal discs and can lead to injury. Consider the hip sockets as hinges and bend forward, keeping the back as straight as possible. This movement will stretch the hamstring muscles at the back of the thighs. Generally, the tightness of these muscles prevents us from touching our toes easily; once the hamstrings are loosened, our flexibility increases enormously.

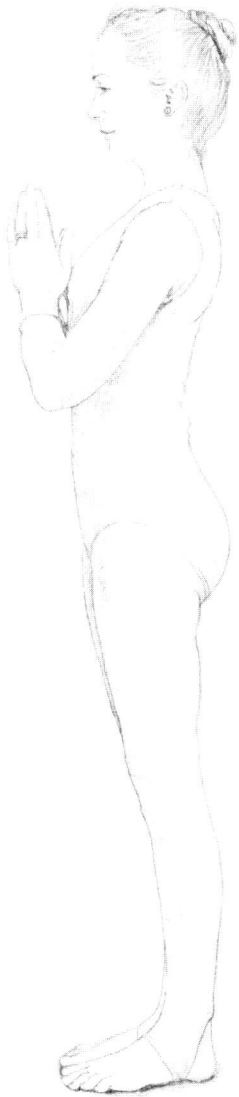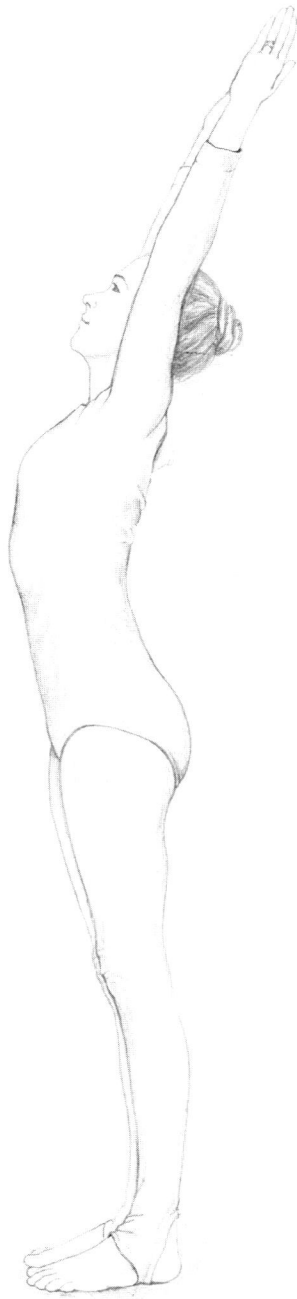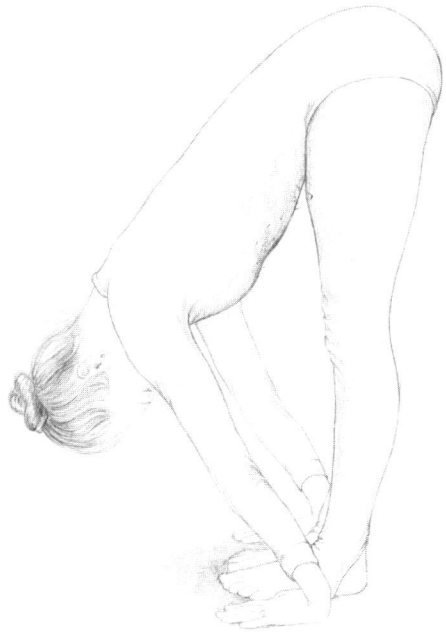

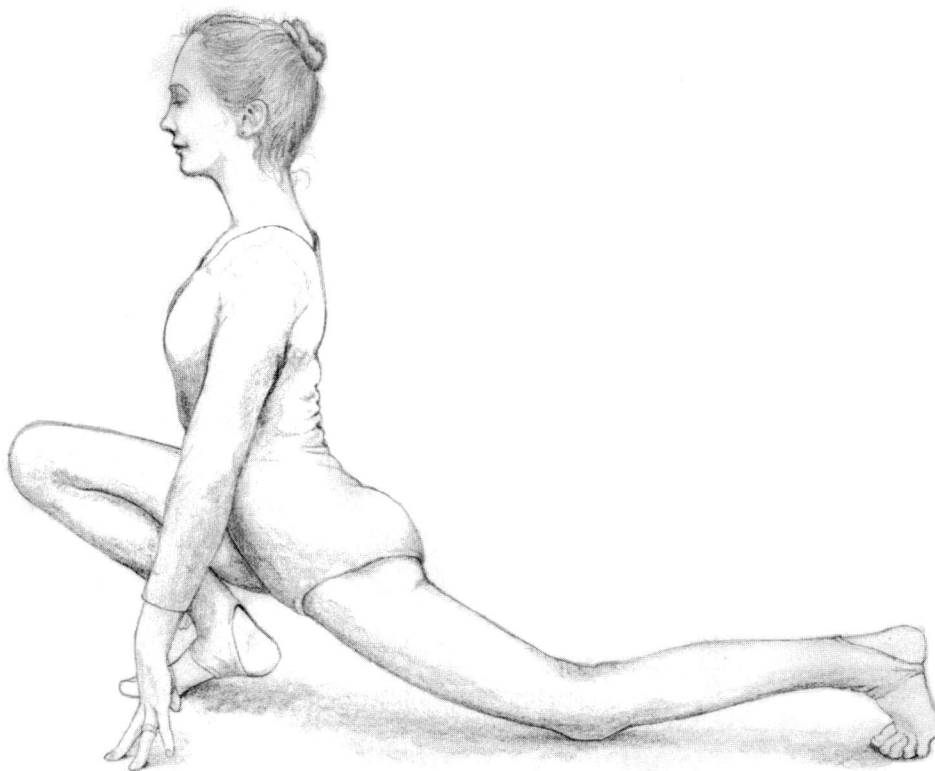

Position 4

- place hands on floor, fingers in line with toes — bending knees, if necessary
- step back with left foot, place knee on ground, curl toes under
- keep hips parallel and lower slowly towards floor, stretching front left thigh
- inhale, come up on fingertips, and lift spinal column
- open chest, draw shoulders down, and lengthen back of head and neck

Position 5

- exhale, bring right foot back beside left foot, feet slightly apart and parallel
- lift buttocks and extend sitting bones toward ceiling to lengthen spine
- keep legs straight, kneecaps lifted, and press heels down towards floor
- press hands into floor, straighten elbows, and lift breastbone towards navel

This position is described in greater detail under *Adho Mukha Svanasana* (Downward Facing Dog Pose).

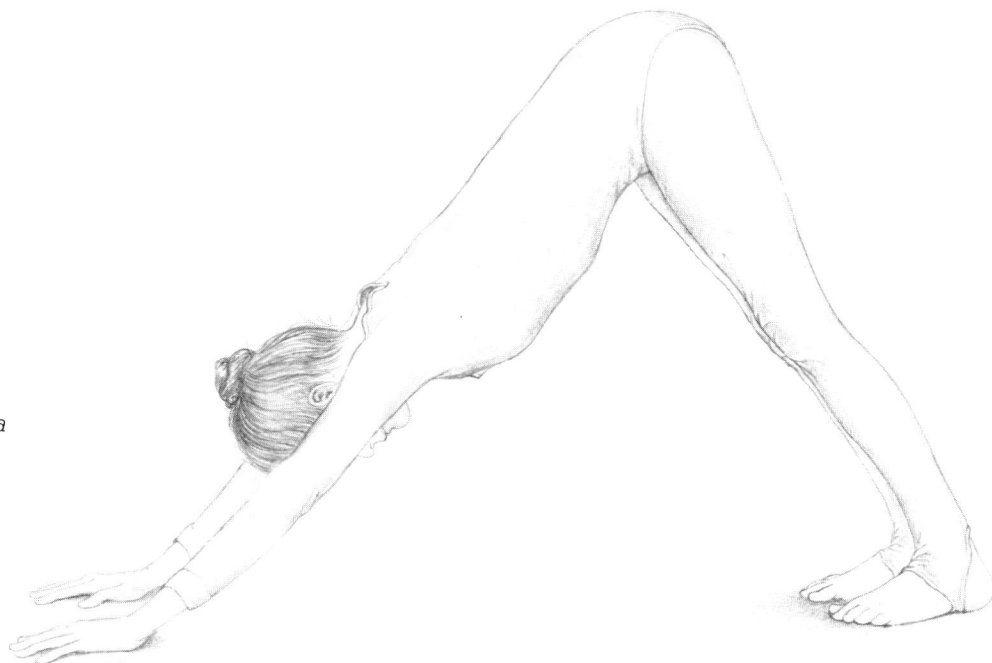

Position 6

- hold breath out, drop knees to floor
- lower chest to floor between hands

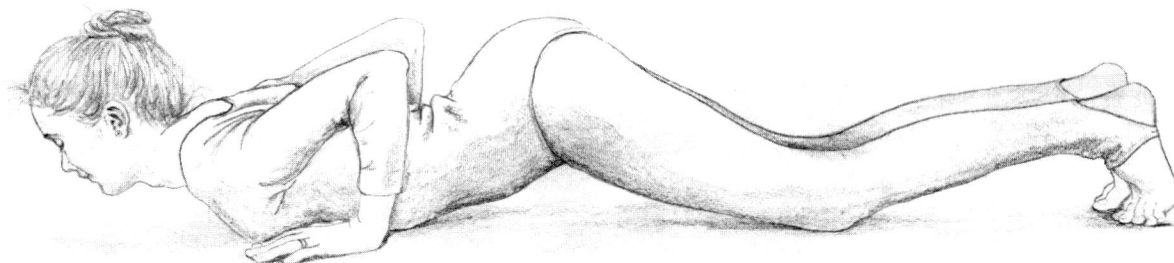

Position 7

- inhale, straighten arms, draw shoulders down, open chest and lift spinal column
- raise thighs off floor, open back of knees and keep buttocks firm to protect lower back

This position is described in greater detail under *Urdhva Mukha Svanasana* (Upward Facing Dog Pose).

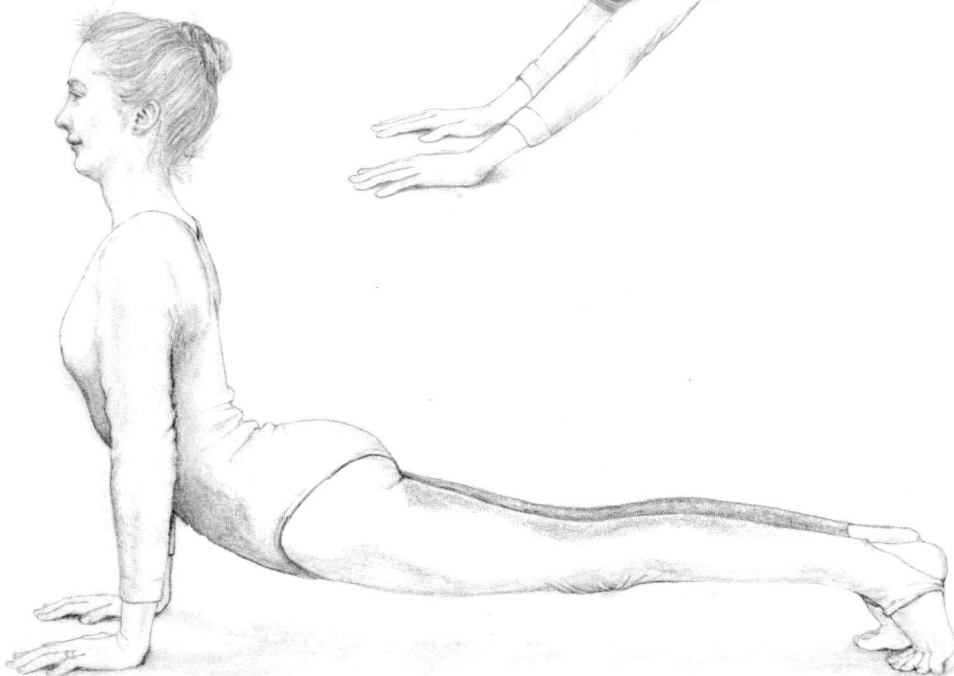

Postion 8

- exhale, lift buttocks high, as in Position 5
- push up from hands to extend spine as much as possible

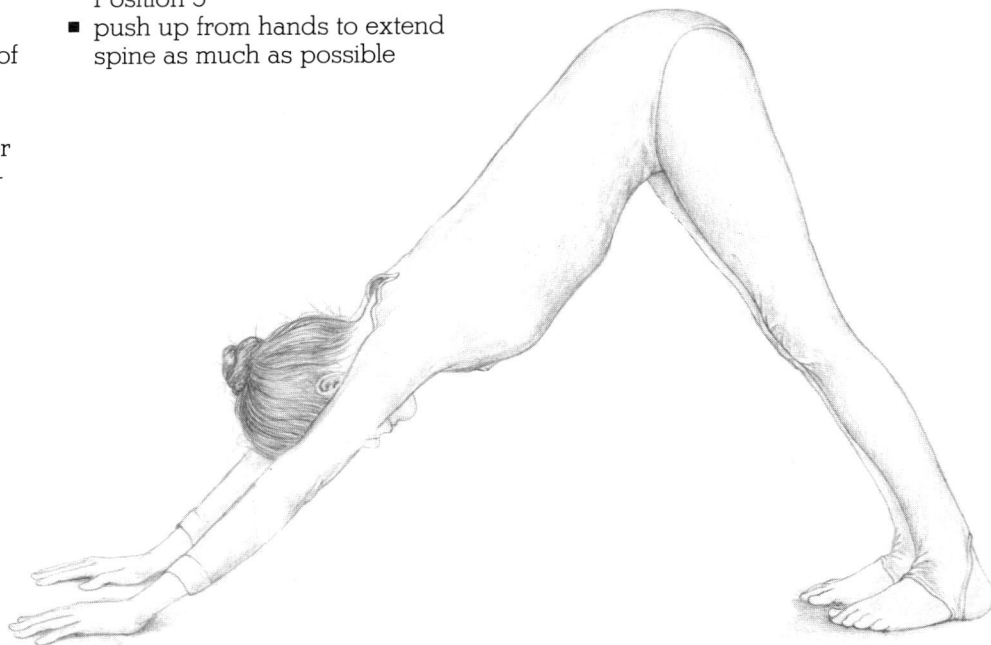

Position 9

- inhale, bring right foot between hands
- exhale, place left knee on floor and lower hips, keeping them parallel
- inhale, come up on fingertips and lift spine as in Position 4

Position 10

- bring left foot forward in line with right foot, keeping feet slightly apart for balance
- straighten legs and lift kneecaps as in Position 3
- release deeper into forward bend on exhalation

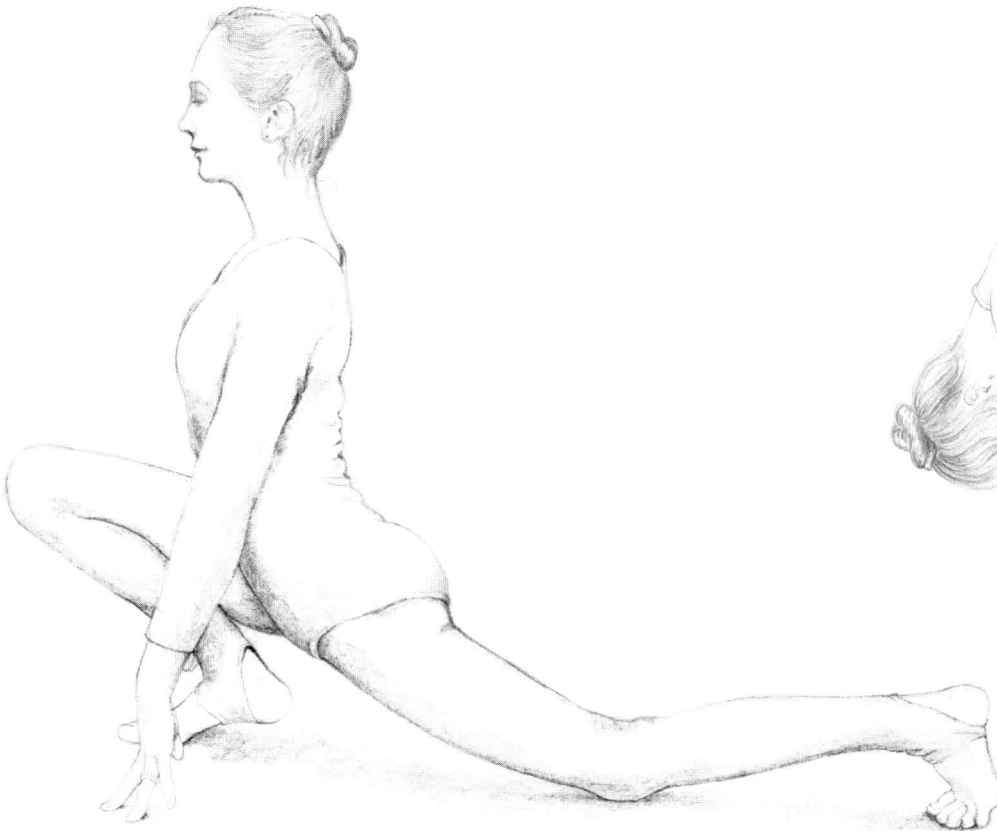

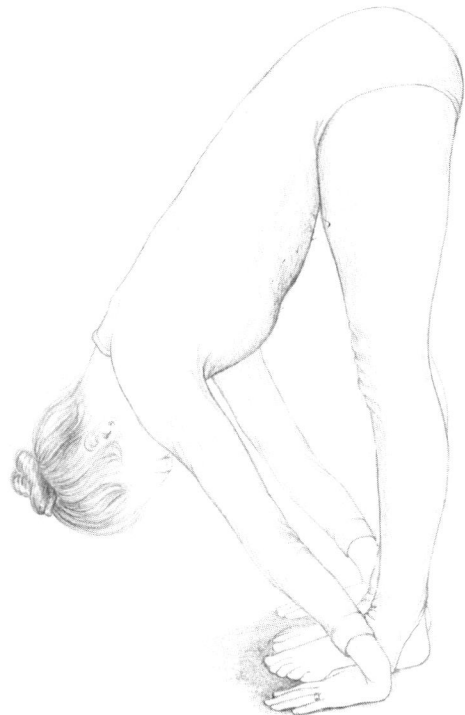

Position 11

- extend arms forward until back is straight
- inhale, raise upper body, using hips as a hinge
- keep kneecaps lifted and buttocks firm
- stretch arms up from armpits, and open upper chest, as in Position 2

Position 12

- exhale, lower arms and bring hands to *namaskar* position, as in Position 1
- soften the eyes, and draw your attention inward
- observe the sensations of change taking place within your body

Positions 1 through 12 constitute *half* of a full round of *Surya Namaskar.* (See Appendix for condensed illustration of the 12 positions.) For the second half of the round, the same movements are repeated with a variation in Positions 4 and 9. In Position 4, the right leg should go to the back, and in Position 9, the left leg should come forward between the hands.

Two halves complete one full round of *Surya Namaskar.* Once the leg changes are learned, counting the number of rounds becomes easy. When the left leg is back you know you are on the first half of the round; when you swing your right leg back, you know you are on the second half.

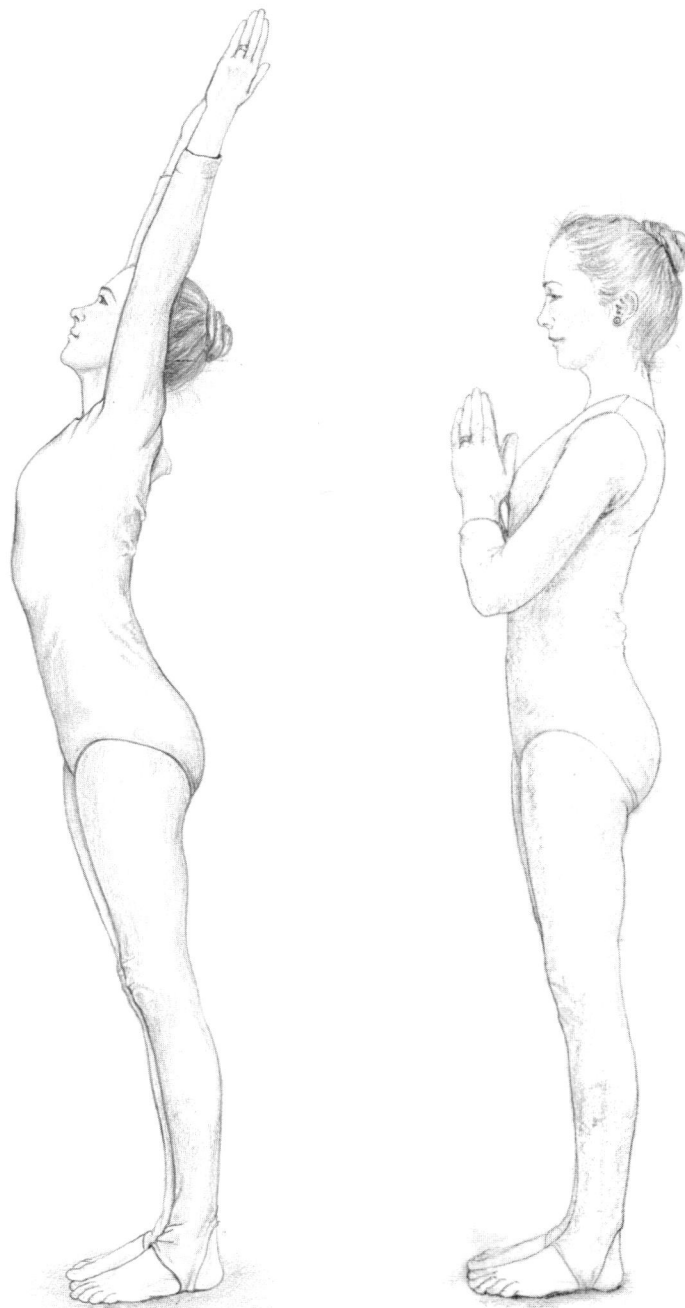

Warming-up Postures

Before attempting the more difficult asanas, it is advisable to prepare the body gradually with some warm-up movements of the pelvis that give a mild stretch to the leg and back muscles and ease the stiffness of the joints. This is particularly important if you have not been exercising regularly. The postures in this chapter focus on the mobility of the pelvis, on warming the major muscles of the legs and back, and on increasing circulation to the spinal column.

The remaining chapters of this book are set forth in a deliberate sequence. The standing poses strengthen the legs and realign the pelvis, thus providing a firm foundation for the spine. The forward bends and backward bends then increase the range of movement of the spine. The spinal twists which follow act as counterposes, returning the spine to a neutral position. The shoulderstand series calms the spinal nerves and gives us an experience of inner harmony. The reclining poses release any physical discomfort generated by our practice. And finally, the relaxation pose encourages us to let go on the mental level as well, and to unite with the inner Self.

KONASANA
(*kona*, angle; right angle pose)

Stand facing a wall, table or ledge with feet parallel and a few inches apart.

- bring hands onto wall at hip-level, and walk feet back until torso is parallel to floor, with arms fully extended, and feet directly under center of hips — forming a right angle between torso and legs
- keep arches lifted, and knees and thighs drawn firmly upwards
- stretch arms and press sitting bones away from wall so that pelvis rotates forward and entire back lengthens
- hold for 1 or 2 minutes, and come up on inhalation

For those with tight hamstrings and lower back problems: place the hands higher on the wall, in order to extend the spine.

Benefits
Konasana is an excellent warm-up with which to begin a daily practice. It lengthens the spine, gives a mild stretch to the hamstrings, and gradually opens the shoulders.

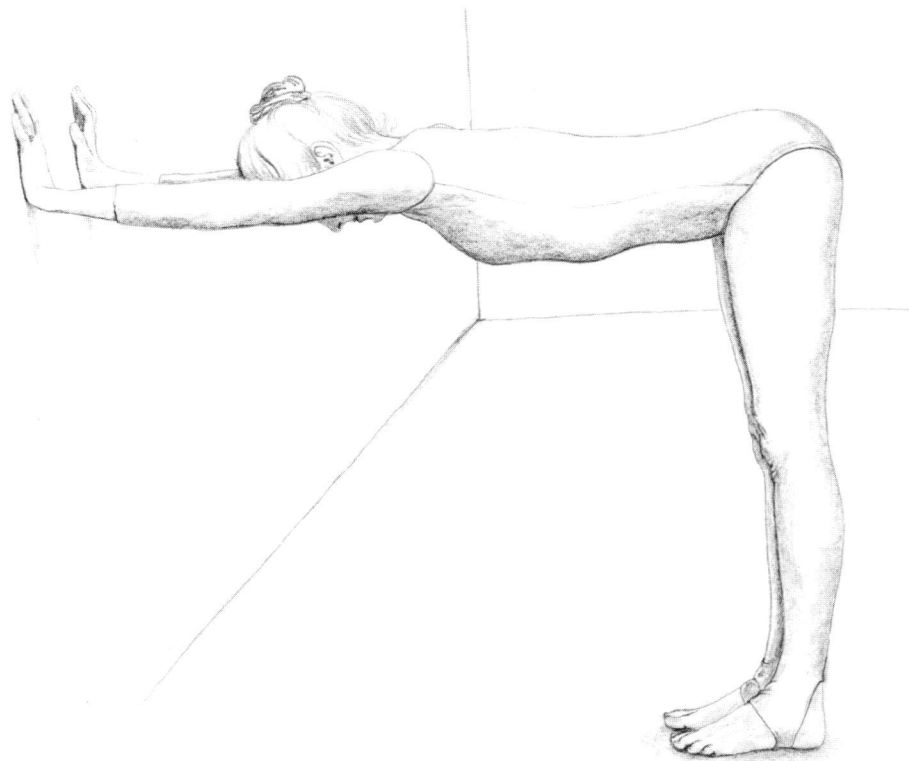

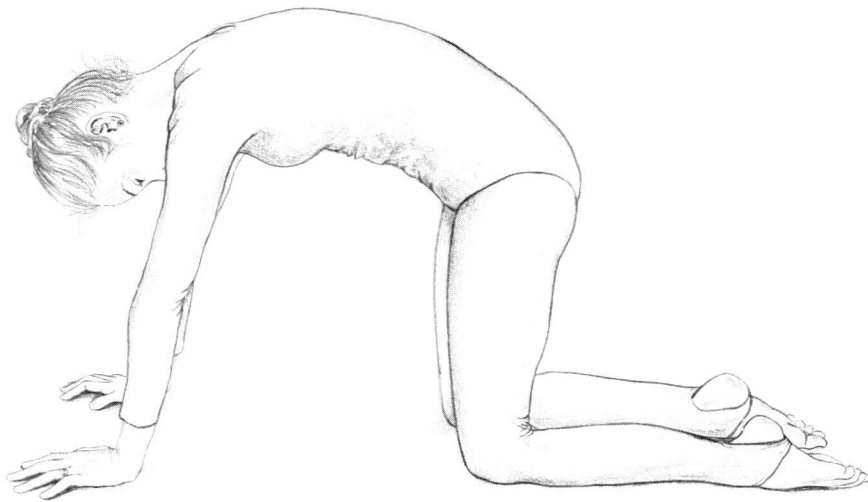

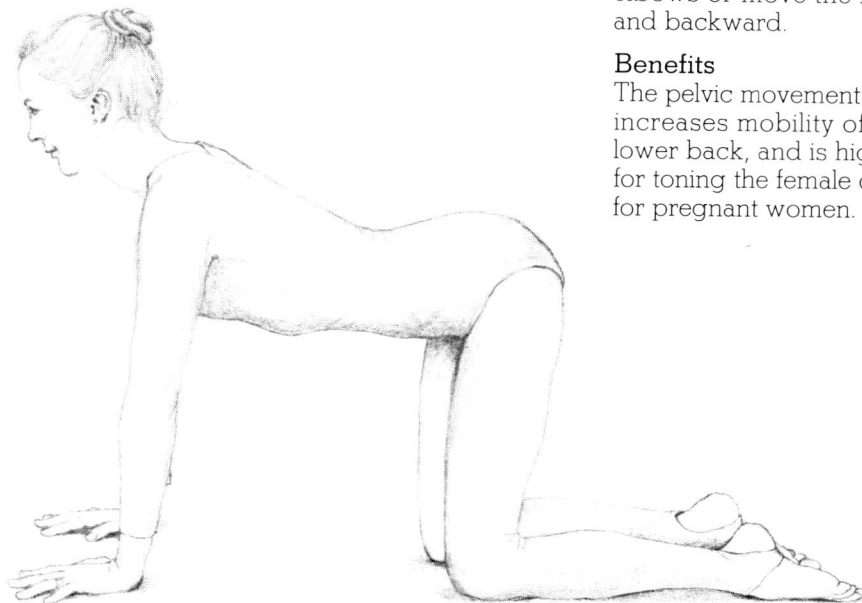

VIDALASANA

(*vidala*, cat; cat pose)

Start from a kneeling position, and bring the hands onto the floor. The hands should be directly under the shoulders about twelve inches apart. The knees should be directly under the hips, just a few inches apart, and the spine extended parallel to the floor.

- on exhalation, move tailbone down towards floor, allowing head to drop and upper back to round
- on inhalation, lift tailbone towards ceiling, so that pelvis rotates forward; open chest, allow upper back to arch and lengthen back of head and neck

Repeat several times, moving only the head and spine. Do not bend the elbows or move the body forward and backward.

Benefits

The pelvic movement in this pose increases mobility of the hips and lower back, and is highly beneficial for toning the female organs and for pregnant women.

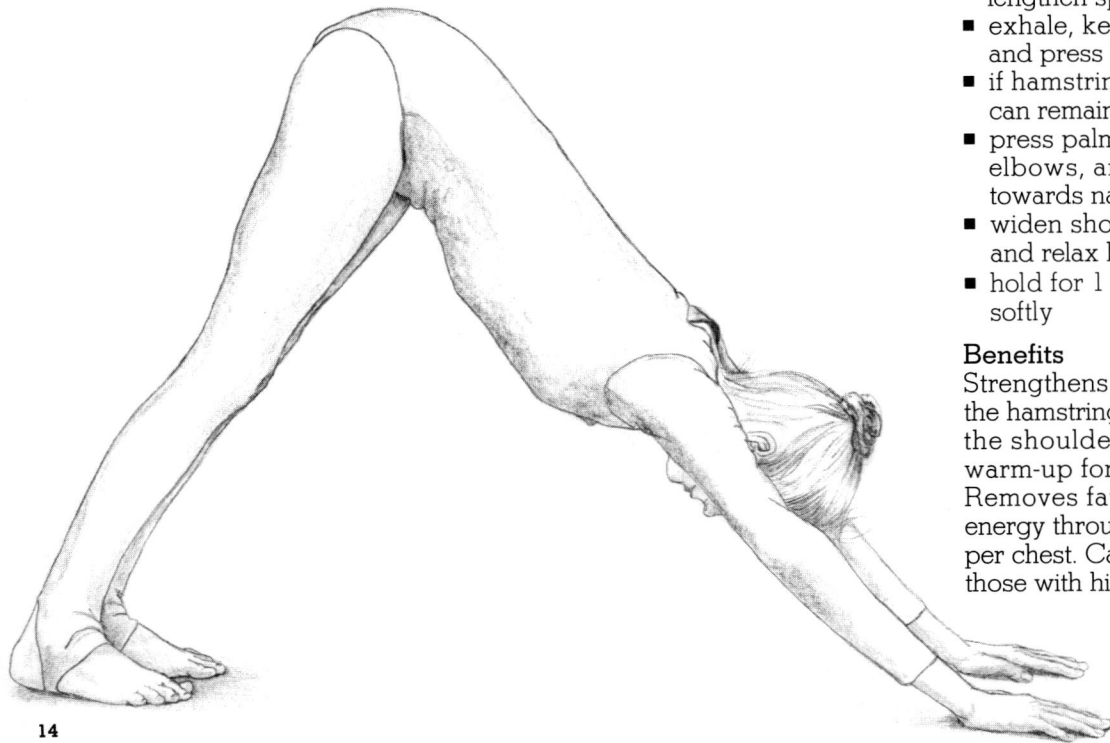

ADHO MUKHA SVANASANA

(*adho*, downward; *mukha*, face; *svana*, dog; downward facing dog pose)

From a kneeling position, bring the hands onto the floor, as for Cat Pose. The hands should be directly under the shoulders, the knees a few inches apart and directly under the hips, and the torso parallel to the floor.

- spread palms on floor, and curl toes under
- exhale, straighten legs, and lift buttocks up
- inhale, lift high onto toes, extend sitting bones toward ceiling to lengthen spine
- exhale, keep kneecaps lifted and press heels towards floor
- if hamstrings are tight, heels can remain slightly off floor
- press palms into floor, straighten elbows, and lift breastbone towards navel
- widen shoulders, lengthen neck, and relax base of throat
- hold for 1 or 2 minutes, breathing softly

Benefits

Strengthens the legs, stretches the hamstrings and spine, and opens the shoulder joints. Excellent warm-up for runners and athletes. Removes fatigue and restores energy through flow of blood to upper chest. Can be practiced safely by those with high blood pressure.

14

DYNAMIC PLOW MOVEMENT

Lie on your back with arms stretched overhead. Beginners can start with hands by the sides, palms pressing down, and bring arms overhead after toes touch floor. Practice on a blanket or carpet to protect the spine. To avoid undue strain, bend knees slightly when raising or lowering legs.

- with a quick rolling movement bring legs overhead and touch toes to floor
- maintaining the momentum, bring legs back to floor, roll torso to forward bend position, and extend arms beyond feet
- bring torso and arms back to reclining position, and repeat cycle several times until movement becomes smooth and even

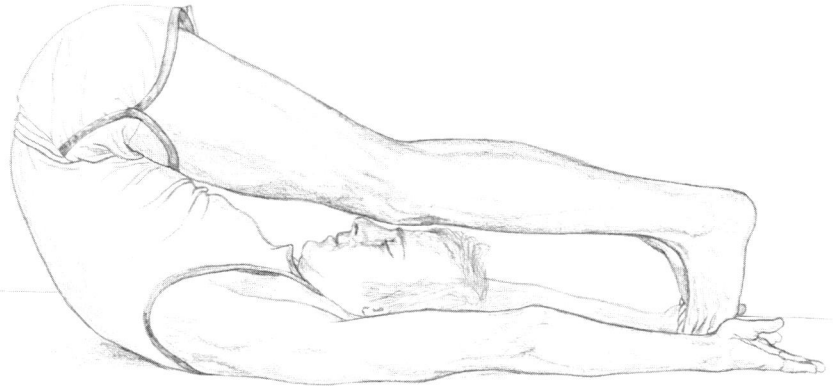

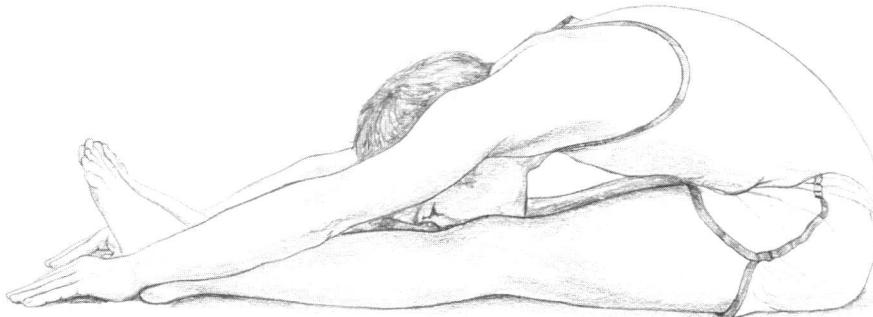

Standing Postures

The standing postures are extremely important for the meditator. These asanas develop the strength and flexibility of the legs and lower back. They help to improve your overall posture, through correct alignment of the spinal column and pelvis. When the spinal column is properly supported by the pelvis, it is possible to sit comfortably for meditation and to maintain the posture for any length of time.

The standing postures provide you with a strong foundation, and with a sense of grounding. They will also strengthen and protect the knees, if you remember to lift your kneecaps whenever the legs are extended, and to keep the center of the knee pointing in the same direction as the foot.

The balancing postures develop a sense of balance, grace and concentration. They help to coordinate mental awareness with movement of the body and bring a finer sensitivity to your physical activity. In order to perform the balancing postures correctly, concentration is essential. This can be acquired by focusing the mind on a point of concentration (a spot on the wall or floor), and sustaining that throughout the pose.

TADASANA

(tada, mountain; mountain pose)

This is the basic standing pose. Come back to it between other standing poses as a quiet resting place.

Stand with the base of the big toes touching, and heels slightly apart.

- lift toes off floor, spread balls of feet, then lower toes to floor
- distribute weight of the body evenly on both feet, and between balls of feet and heels
- draw up calf muscles, lift kneecaps, and draw up thigh muscles both inner and outer
- firm outer hips and draw tailbone deeper into body, thus extending lower back
- open upper chest, and keep diaphragm soft and wide
- head and neck balance on upper spinal column, with eyes soft and jaw relaxed
- on inhalation, firm legs and feel whole spinal column lifting upward through crown of head
- on exhalation, maintain lift of spinal column as shoulders and arms release downwards
- hold pose for 1 minute, breathing quietly

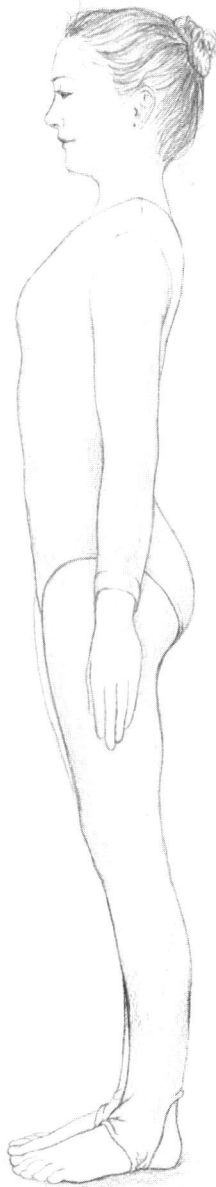

If you check your posture sideways in a mirror, there should be a straight line running from the center of the ears, down through the center of the shoulders, hips and knees to the ankle bones. There should be a slight tilt of the pelvis to maintain the natural curve of the lumbar spine. If the lumbar is either overarched or overflattened, there will be constant pressure on the vertebrae and discs. In all your poses, think of lengthening the spinal column, not of flattening the back, so that you create maximum space between the vertebrae and thus maintain a healthy spine.

Benefits

Strengthens the legs, and develops awareness of balance and correct posture. The principles of alignment learned in *Tadasana* can be applied to all other poses.

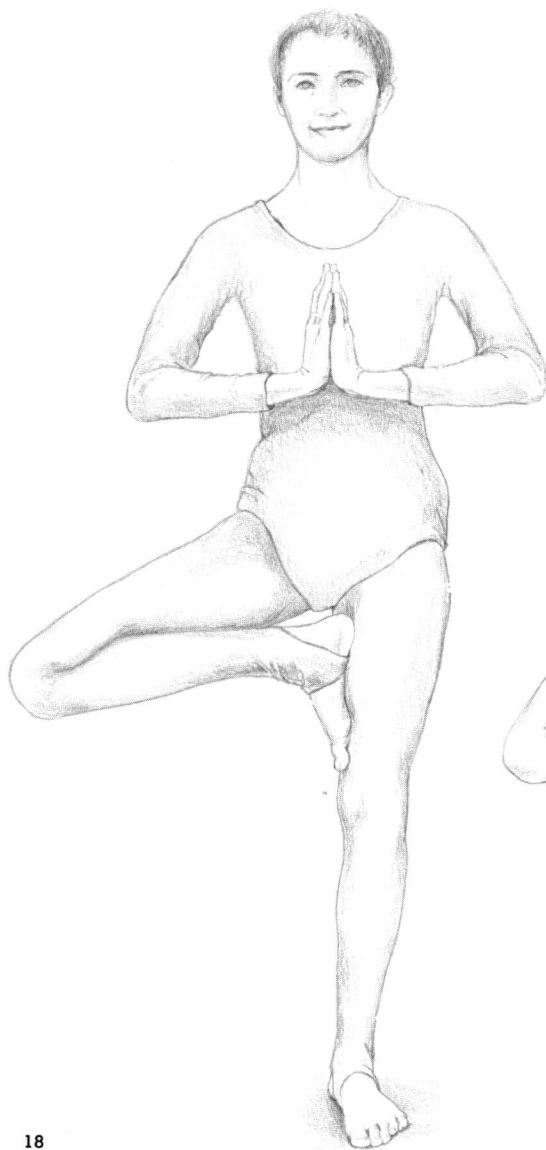

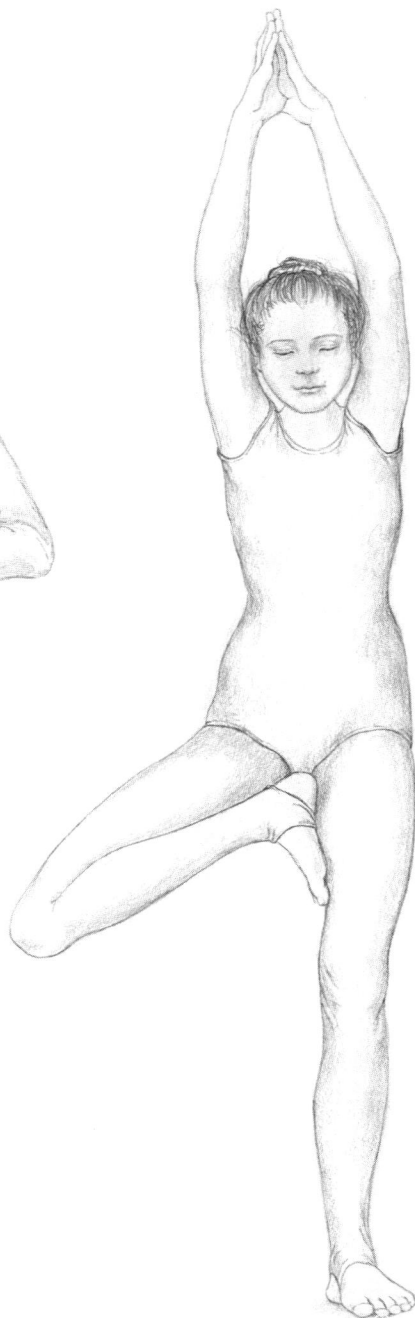

VRIKSHASANA

(*vriksha*, tree; tree pose)

Stand in *Tadasana* with feet together and arms by the sides. If balance is difficult, practice this pose with the back against a wall.

VARIATION 1

- focus eyes on a point directly ahead to help maintain balance
- turn right thigh out, raise foot, and take hold of right ankle
- place sole of foot firmly on inner left thigh, with heel as high as possible
- keep both hips facing directly forward, and extend inner right thigh towards bent knee
- bring palms together in front of chest (*namaskar* position), with shoulders widening, and forearms parallel to floor
- keep thigh of standing leg very firm, and continue to lift from base of spine
- hold for half a minute, and repeat on other side

VARIATION 2

When balance becomes easy, try this variation for a more dynamic lift.

- raise arms overhead, place palms together, and straighten elbows

Benefits

Vrikshasana tones and strengthens the legs and gives a sense of balance. It is excellent for steadying the mind and developing concentration.

TRIKONASANA
(*trikona, triangle; triangle pose*)

Stand with the feet about 3 to 3½ feet apart; the correct distance is the length of your own leg.

- turn left foot in 30° and right foot out 90°
- for proper alignment, heel of right foot should be in line with arch of left foot
- inhale, raise arms to shoulder level, extending from middle of back to fingertips
- lift kneecaps, and make sure that center of right knee points directly towards right foot — this will protect inner knee from injury
- exhale, bend from hip joint, extending torso sideways to the right, in line with legs
- place right hand on ankle or shin, and extend left arm vertically, with palm of left hand facing forward
- lengthen spinal column and open chest, so that ribcage faces directly forward
- turn head towards ceiling, tucking chin slightly
- hold for a half a minute, breathing normally

Return to standing position, and repeat to other side.

Benefits
Trikonasana is an intense lateral stretch which opens the chest and hips, and strengthens the legs.

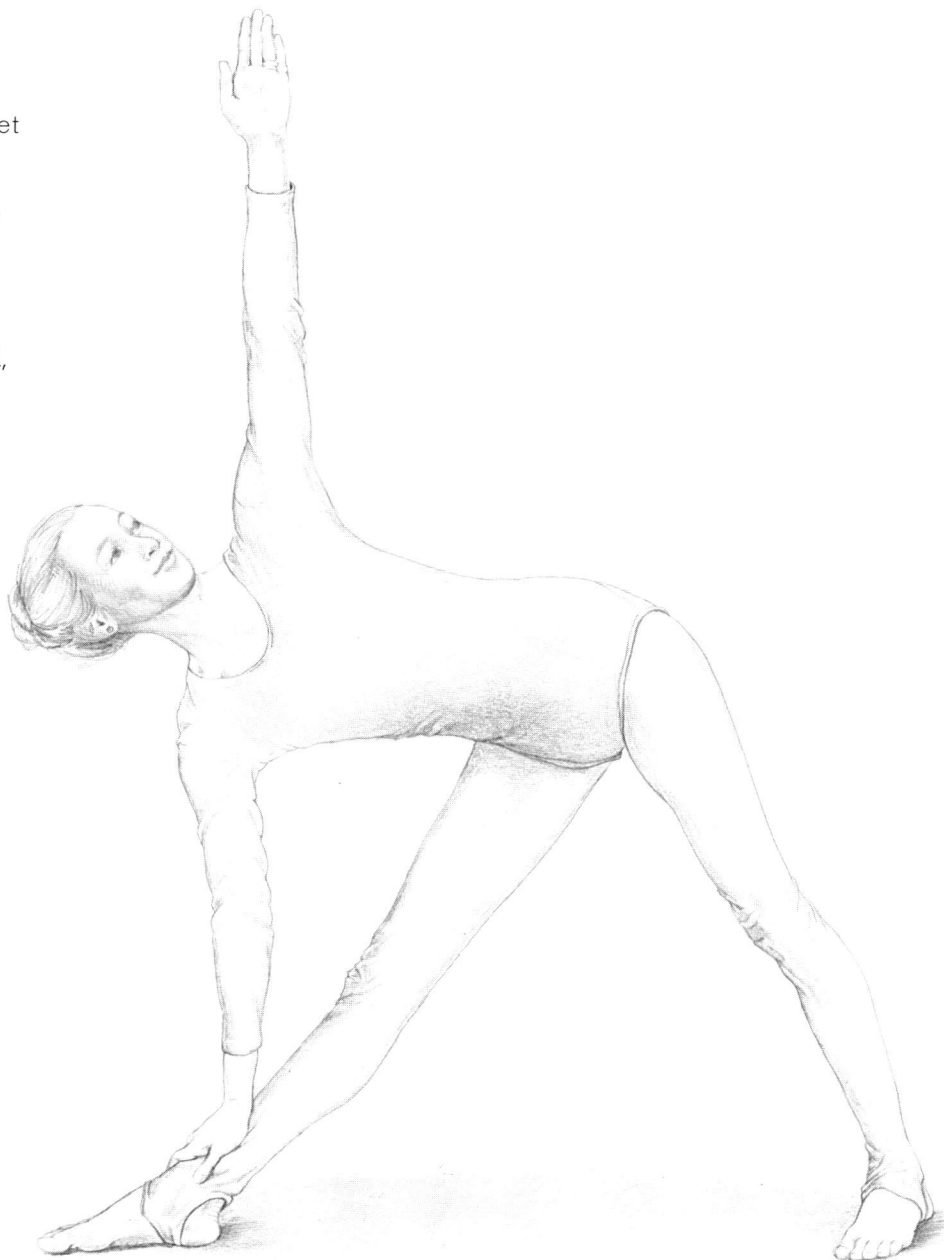

PARSVAKONASANA

(parsva, side; *kona*, angle; side angle pose)

Stand with feet approximately 4 to 4½ feet apart, about one foot wider than in *Trikonasana*.

- turn right foot in 30° and left foot out 90°
- for proper alignment, heel of left foot should be in line with arch of right foot
- inhale, raise arms to shoulder level, extending from middle of back to fingertips
- exhale, bend left knee until thigh is parallel to floor, and knee is directly over heel
- inhale, lift spinal column, and stretch back through right leg
- exhale, bend from hip joint, extending torso sideways over left thigh
- place left hand on floor by left ankle—or place a block under hand if you cannot reach floor easily
- extend right arm over right ear with palm down, so that upper side of body stretches from right foot to right fingertips

- turn head towards ceiling, and lengthen back of neck, keeping eyes soft
- hold for half a minute, breathing normally

Return to standing position, and repeat to other side.

Benefits

This posture gives an intense lateral stretch, and also strengthens the legs and loosens the hip joints.

Caution

Do not let the bent knee collapse inwards, as this puts great strain on the inner knee. Keep the bent knee directly over the center of the heel.

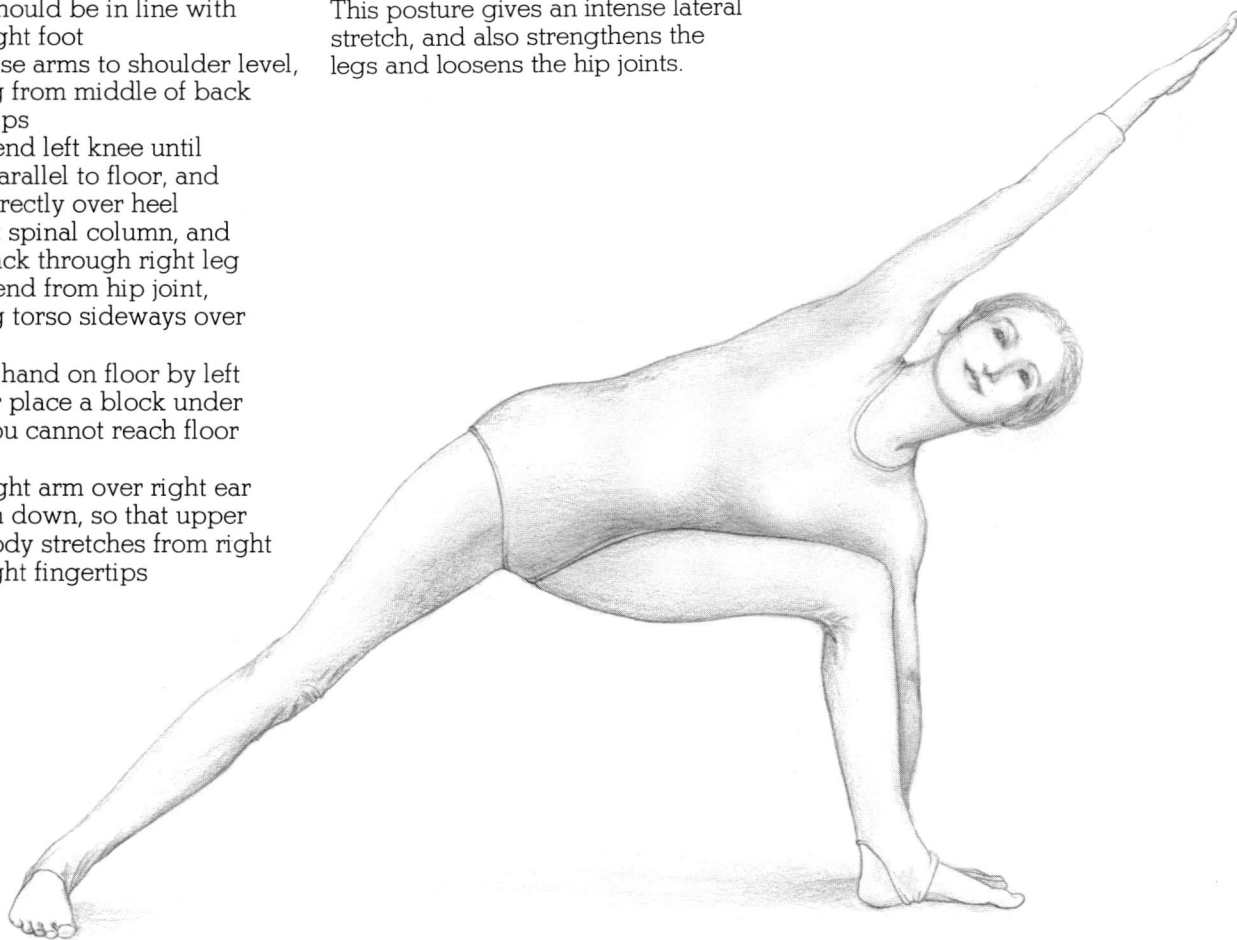

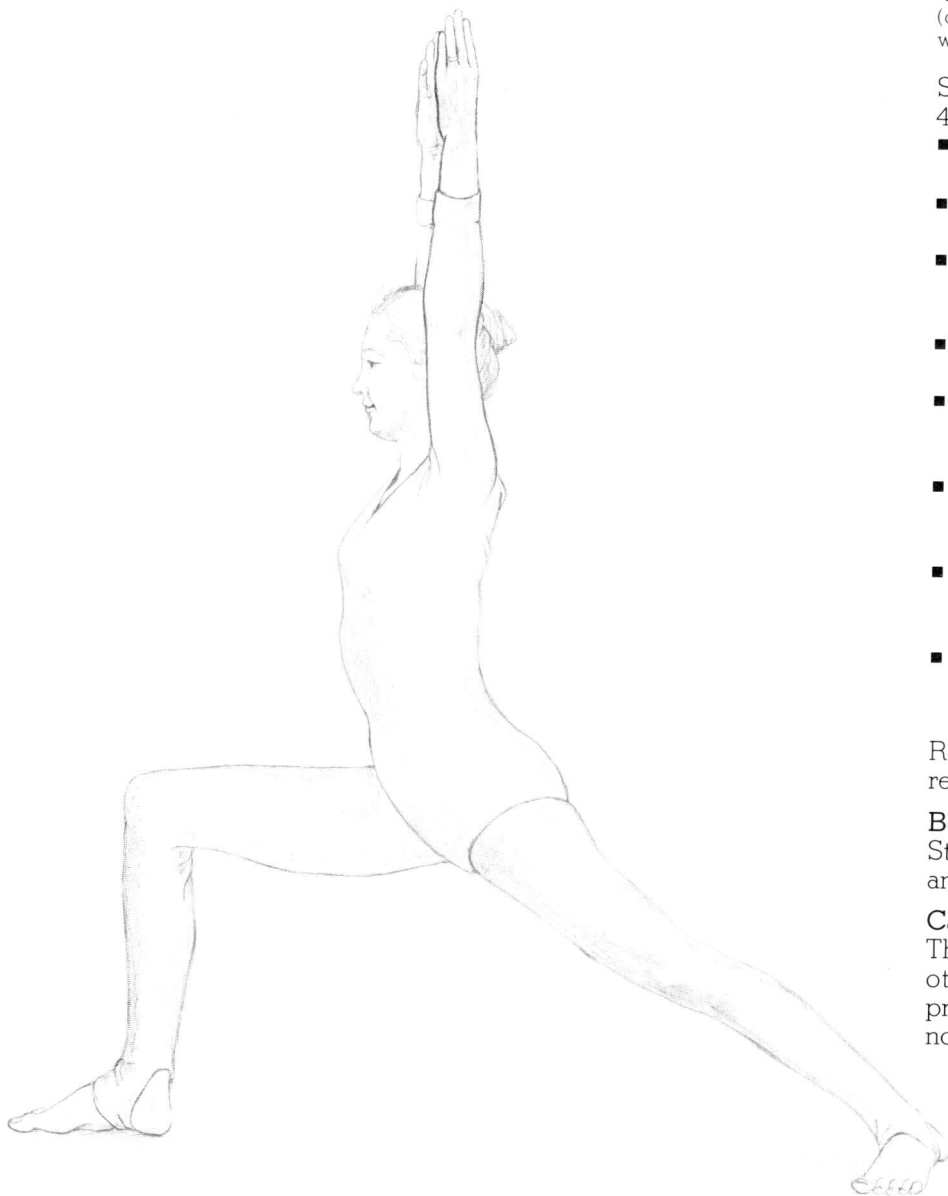

VIRABHADRASANA I

(dedicated to *Virabhadra*, a warrior; warrior pose)

Stand with feet approximately 4 to 4½ feet apart.

- turn left foot in 60° and right foot out 90°
- heel of right foot should be in line with arch of left foot
- inhale, raise arms overhead, palms facing each other, and elbows straight
- exhale, turn torso to face right leg, so that hips are parallel
- inhale, straighten left leg and knee, lifting upwards from base of spine
- exhale, bend right knee until thigh is parallel to floor, and knee is directly over heel
- keep shoulder girdle directly over center of front hip to avoid compression in lower back
- hold for half a minute, breathing softly, and release tension from neck, throat and shoulders

Return to standing position, and repeat to the other side.

Benefits
Strengthens the legs, opens the chest and relieves stiffness in the shoulders.

Caution
Those with high blood pressure or other heart conditions should practice this pose with hands on hips, not overhead.

VIRABHADRASANA II
(dedicated to *Virabhadra*, a warrior; warrior pose)

Stand with feet approximately 4 to 4½ feet apart.

- turn left foot in 30° and right foot out 90°
- heel of right foot should be in line with arch of left foot
- inhale, raise arms to shoulder level, extending from middle of back to fingertips
- exhale, bend right knee until thigh is parallel to floor and knee is directly over heel
- stretch left arm towards left hand, so that crown of head stays directly over tailbone, and stretch back through left leg
- turn head and look softly at right hand
- hold for half a minute, maintaining strength in legs and lift of spinal column

Return to standing position and repeat to other side.

Benefits
Strengthens the legs and lower back, and tones the abdominal organs.

Caution
Do not let the bent knee collapse inwards, as this puts great strain on the inner knee. Keep the bent knee directly over the center of the heel.

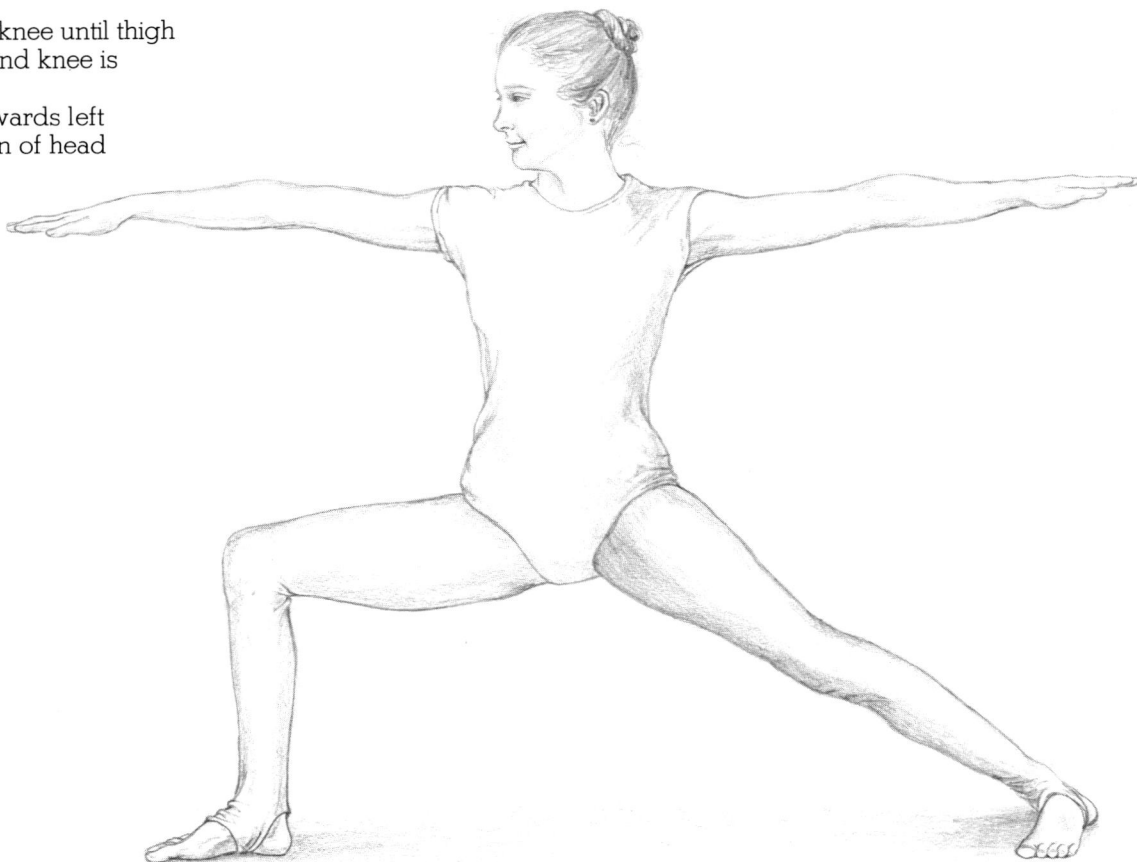

UTTANASANA

(ut, intense; tan, stretch; posture which gives an intense stretch)

This pose is very soothing and relaxing, and can be practiced in between other standing poses to eliminate fatigue.

VARIATION 1

For beginning students: stand with feet parallel, and a few inches apart, so that the ankles are directly under the center of the hips.

- place hands on hips
- inhale, draw knees and inner thighs firmly upwards, and lift from base of spine
- exhale, bend from hip joints and lengthen front of torso until parallel to floor
- allow back to round gently, take hold of elbows, and let head hang freely
- keep knees and thighs lifted, but release abdomen and sides of waist
- hold for half a minute, and come up slowly with hands on hips

This variation can also be practiced with the buttocks resting against a wall, and the feet about 12 to 15 inches away from the wall, so that the entire weight of the body is supported by a wall.

Benefits

Uttanasana slows down the heart and calms the mind. Besides stretching the hamstrings and strengthening the legs, it tones the abdominal organs, and helps to relieve stomach pains and menstrual cramps.

Caution

For those with low blood pressure, remember to come out of the pose very slowly to avoid dizziness.

VARIATION 2

For more advanced students: stand with the feet together — the big toes should be touching but the heels may be slightly apart.

- inhale, raise arms overhead, with palms facing each other and elbows straight
- exhale, bend from hip joints, and lengthen back of arms and front of torso until fingers touch floor
- bring chest toward thighs, and place hands beside feet, with fingers pointing directly forward
- keep knees and thighs actively lifting, but soften abdomen and let head hang freely
- hold for half a minute, and come up by extending arms overhead and lengthening torso

(See Position 3, page 5).

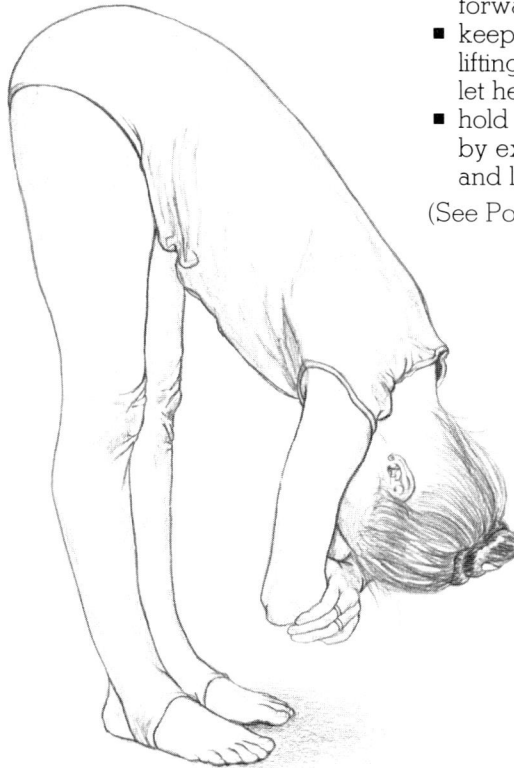

23

PARSVOTTANASANA

(*parsva*, side; *ut*, intense; *tan*, stretch; an intense stretch of the side of the body)

Stand with the feet about 3 to 3½ feet apart; the correct distance is the length of your own leg.

- turn left foot in 60° and right foot out 90°
- heel of right foot should be in line with arch of left foot

- bring hands together behind back, fingers pointing upward, and palms together as in *namaskar* position
- if you cannot bring hands into *namaskar*, then cross forearms behind back and hold elbows
- exhale, turn torso to face right leg, so that hips are parallel
- inhale, lift from base of spine, open upper chest and let head drop back
- exhale, bend from hip joints and extend center of chest over right thigh
- lift elbows toward ceiling to open shoulders and chest
- keep both legs straight with knees and thighs drawing firmly upwards
- hold for half a minute, breathing softly

Return to standing position and repeat to other side.

Benefits
Helps to correct round shoulders. Strengthens and tones abdominal organs. Hips and legs are also strengthened.

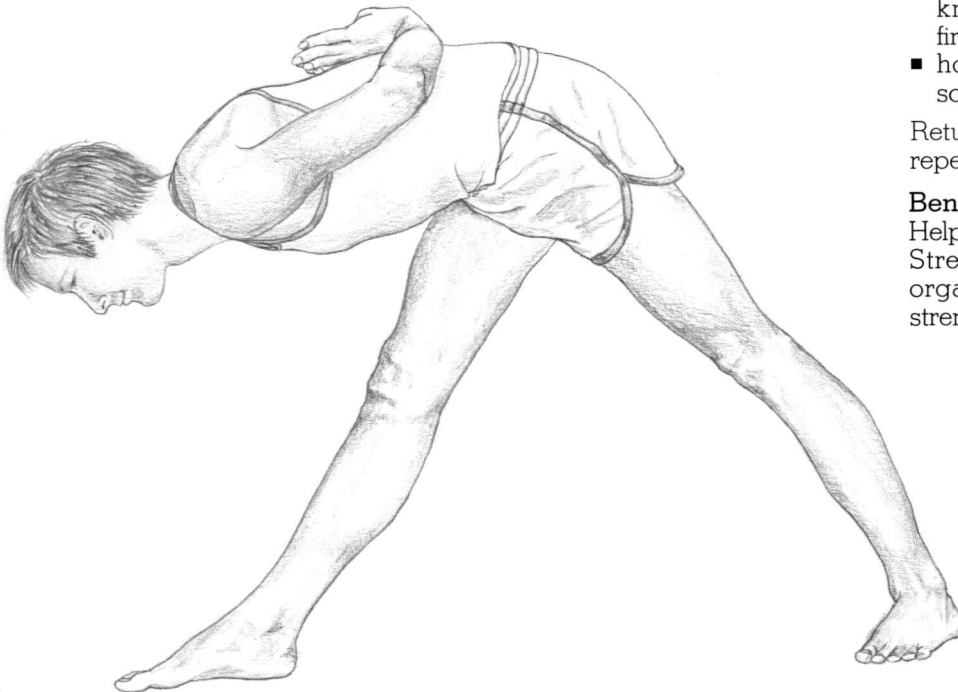

ARDHA CHANDRASANA

(*ardha*, half; *chandra*, moon; half-moon pose)

This pose can be practiced against a wall until the balance is secure enough to try in the center of the room.

Stand with feet about 3 to 3½ feet apart and move into *Trikonasana* (Triangle Pose). If you are using the wall for support, the left foot should be parallel to the wall, and the left hip resting against the wall. Pause for

a few moments in *Trikonasana*, until you feel the quietness and stability of the pose.

- exhale, bend left knee, placing left hand on floor about 12 to 15 inches forward of left foot—if hamstrings are tight, you may need a block or other support under left hand
- inhale, draw weight forward over left foot
- exhale, straighten left leg, and raise right leg until it is in line with outer right hip
- lift left kneecap and inner thigh, and open right hip towards ceiling, but keep right knee and foot pointing forward
- bring arms into a vertical line and extend from middle of back to fingertips, opening upper chest

so that ribcage faces directly forward

- for beginners, eyes can be focused on floor or straight ahead to help with balance
- for more flexible students, when balance is steady, turn head towards ceiling, tucking chin slightly
- hold for half a minute, maintaining strength of legs and softness of breath

Return to standing position and repeat to other side.

Benefits

Creates freedom and openness in chest and pelvis, and is helpful for those with sciatica and other lower back problems.

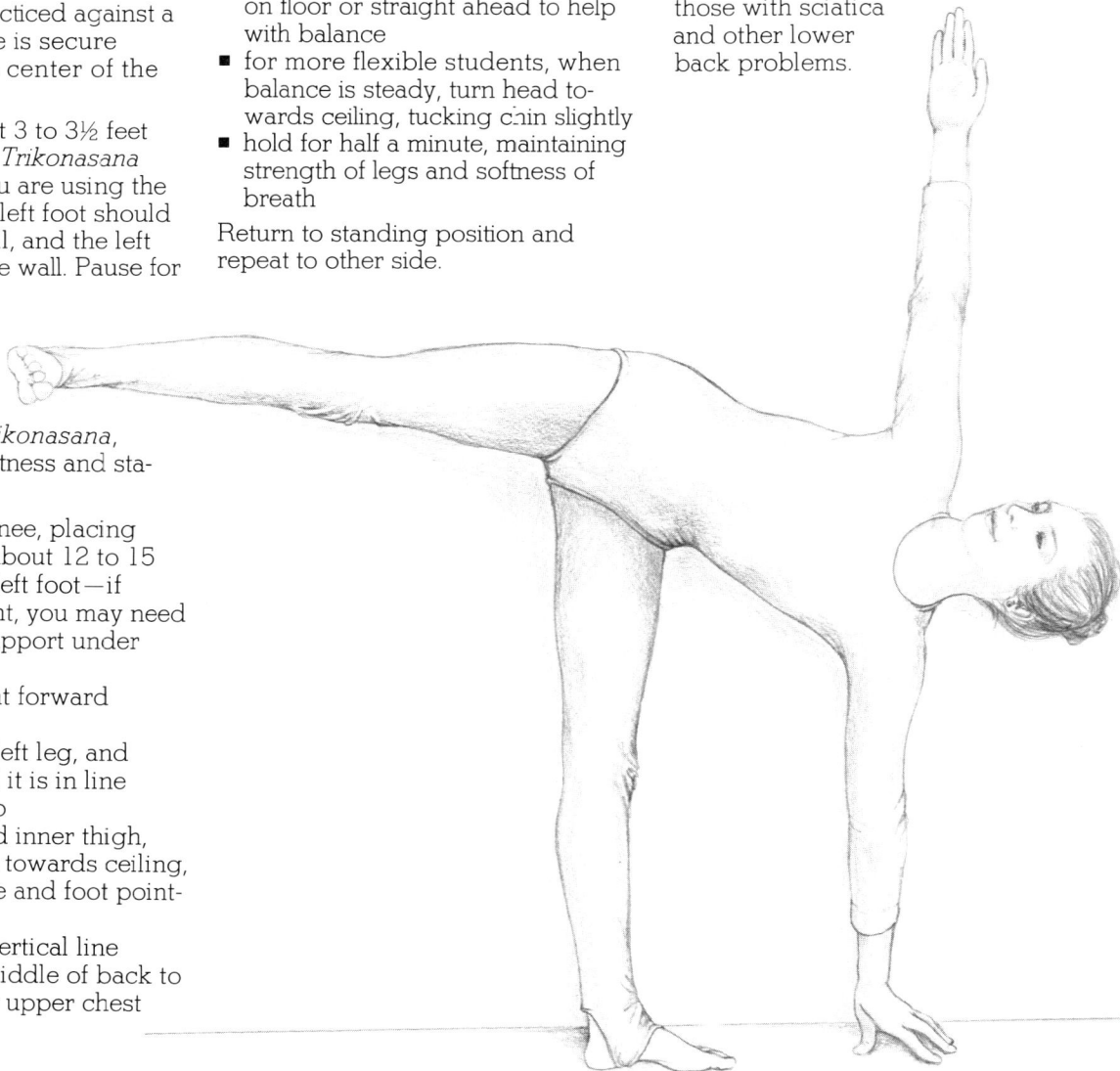

PRASARITA PADOTTANASANA

(*prasarita*, spread; *pada*, foot; *ut*, intense;
tan, stretch; pose where feet are spread wide
to give an intense stretch)

Stand with the feet 4 to 5 feet
apart, and hands on the hips, making
sure that the feet are parallel.

- inhale, draw knees and thighs
  firmly upward, and lift from base of
  spine
- exhale, bend forward from hip
  joints and lengthen front of
  torso
- if hands do not easily reach
  floor, bring hands onto shins
- otherwise, place hands on floor
  in line between feet and shoulder-
  width apart
- inhale, straighten arms, and roll
  sitting bones towards ceiling to
  arch the back, with head
  looking up
- exhale, bend elbows, bring
  chest towards thighs, allowing
  back to round gently
- lift shoulder blades towards waist
  and stretch back of arms towards
  elbows, so that head hangs freely
- for flexible students, head will
  touch floor — at this stage,
  move feet closer together so
  that crown of head barely
  touches floor
- hold for a half a minute, breathing
  softly
- inhale, straighten arms, lengthen
  front of torso, bring hands on hips
  and return to standing position

Benefits
Stretches the hamstrings and the
inner thighs, and gives some of the
benefits of inverted poses because of
the flow of blood to the head.

Caution
If you feel pain or weakness at the
inner knees, bring the feet closer
together, and lift the inner thighs.

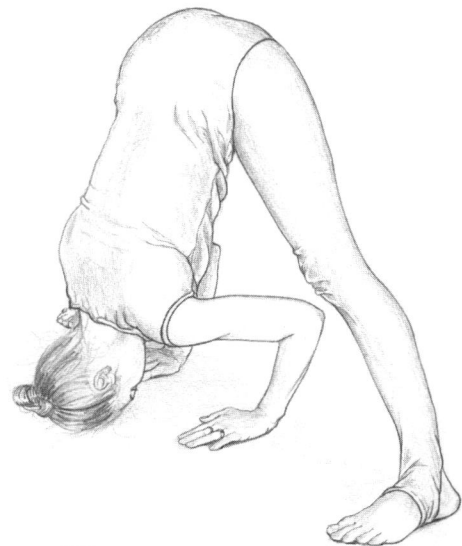

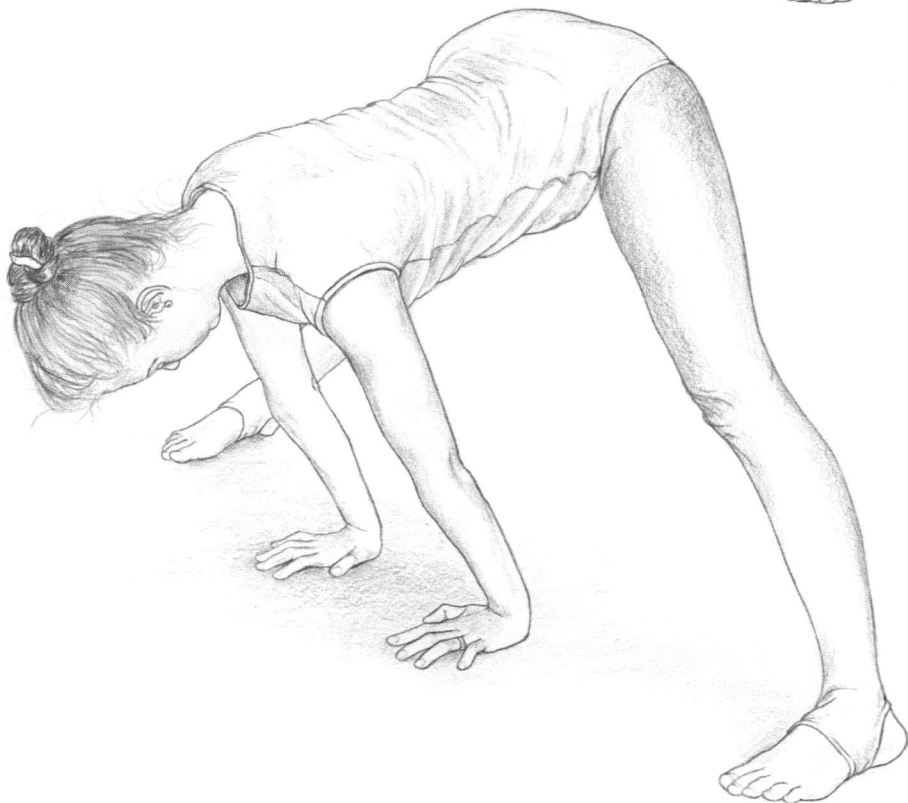

26

PADANGUSTHASANA
(*pada*, foot; *angustha*, big toe; posture holding big toe)

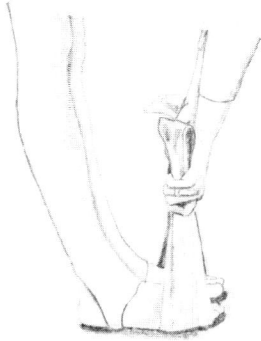

Stand with feet parallel, and a few inches apart, so that the ankles are directly under the hips.

- inhale, draw knees and inner thighs firmly upwards, and lift from base of spine
- exhale, bend from hip joints and lengthen front of torso
- take hold of big toes with second and third fingers, or use a strap around feet if hands do not reach floor easily
- keep arms fully extended, and roll sitting bones towards ceiling to make the back concave
- maintain concave back, lifting thighs and extending spine, moving deeper into pose with each cycle of breath
- on exhalation, bend elbows out to side, bring chest towards thighs, with back gently rounded, and let head hang freely (omit this stage if using a strap)
- hold final position until mind becomes quiet, then come up slowly on inhalation

Benefits
Stretches the legs, lengthens the back, and tones the abdominal organs.

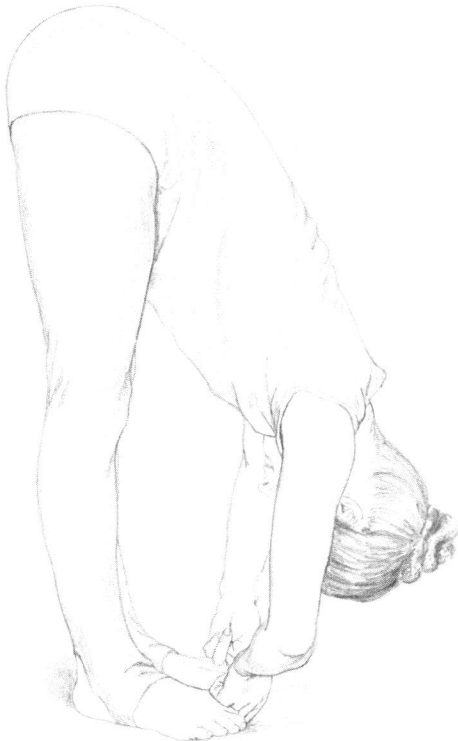

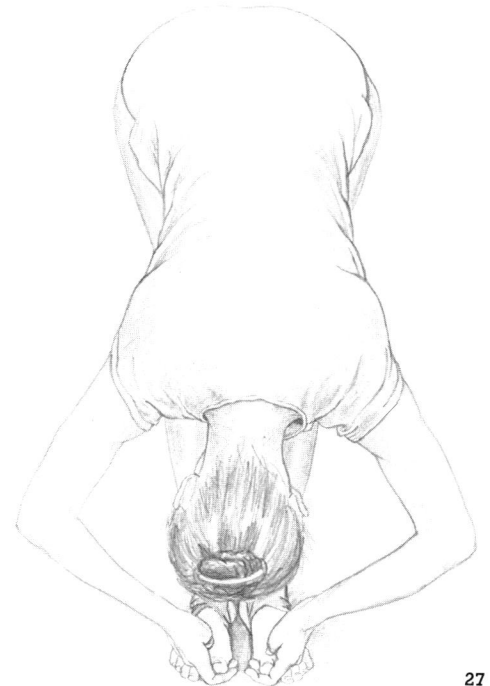

Sitting Postures

The sitting postures in this chapter provide the ideal preparation for a good meditation posture. One of the first problems we confront when beginning the practice of meditation is our inability to sit comfortably in a cross-legged position. The distractions of aching knees, ankles, and back often prevent us from turning our attention within. A cross-legged sitting posture is not natural for most Westerners, yet the yogic texts consider it essential for anyone wishing to advance in meditation.

The ability to sit comfortably in one of the cross-legged postures recommended by Swami Muktananda (*Sukhasana, Swastikasana, Ardha Padmasana* or *Padmasana*) is primarily a matter of loosening the joints of the ankles, knees and hips. This can be accomplished through regular practice of the sitting postures in this chapter. In particular, *Virasana* develops the flexibility of the knees and ankles, and *Baddha Konasana*, the openness of the hips. When both of these asanas have been mastered, one can begin to sit in *Ardha Padmasana* or *Padmasana*.

DANDASANA
(*danda*, stick; stick pose)

This is the basic sitting pose — you can return to this pose as a resting place between other sitting poses.

Sit on the floor with legs outstretched and feet together. Place a blanket underneath the sitting bones, so that the pelvis is tilted slightly forward.

- extend legs, lift kneecaps, and keep knees and toes pointing toward ceiling
- press hands into floor beside hips, draw shoulders down, and lift spine
- center of shoulders should balance directly over center of hips
- breathe softly, and maintain lift of spine and strength of legs
- hold for half a minute

VARIATION
If the hamstrings are very tight, you can hold the feet with a strap, arms fully extended, to help lift the pelvis and spine.

Benefits
Stretches the hamstrings and improves sitting posture.

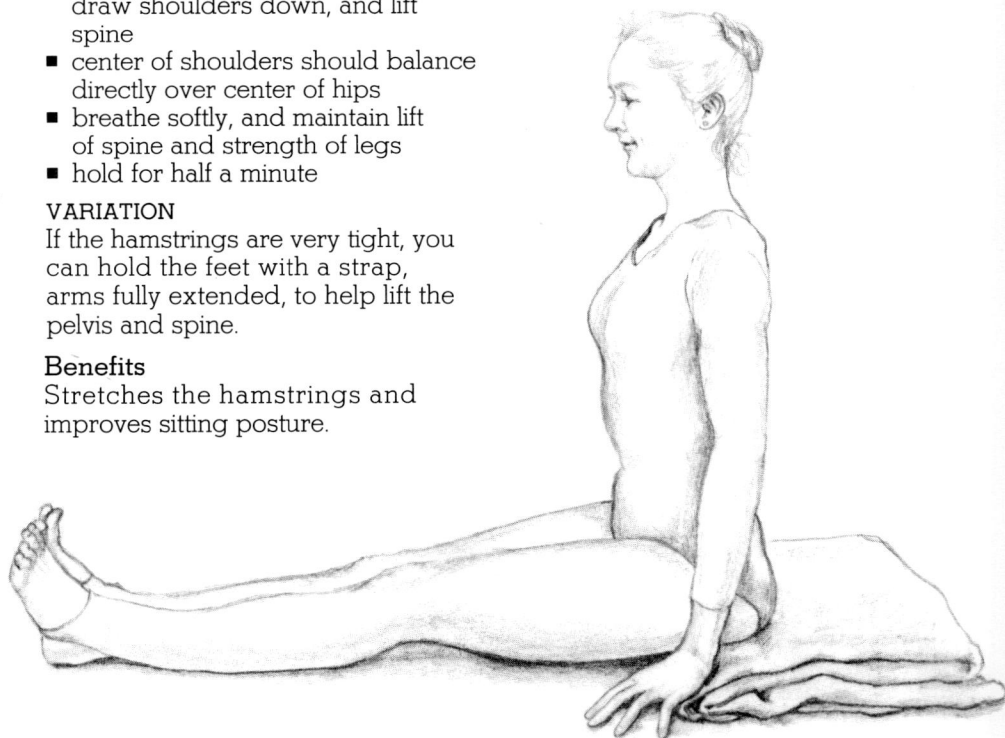

VIRASANA

(*vira*, hero; hero pose)

Sit on the heels with knees together and back erect.

- come to a kneeling position, keep knees together, but spread feet body-width apart
- lower pelvis to rest on floor in between feet — if knees (or ankles) are stiff or painful, place a blanket or cushion under buttocks to a comfortable height
- feet should be alongside hips, not under hips, with toes pointing back and tops of feet resting on floor
- inhale, interlock fingers, raise arms overhead, with elbows straight, and press palms toward ceiling to lengthen spine
- exhale, lower arms, change interlock of fingers, and raise arms overhead again
- hold pose for 1 or 2 minutes altogether

Benefits

Virasana improves the circulation of the legs and is a remedy for varicose veins. Regular practice for several months will help correct flat feet. For the meditator, this is an essential pose for developing the health and flexibility of the knees. *Virasana* aids digestion, and is the only pose which can be practiced immediately after eating.

Caution

If you experience pain in the knee, place a small rolled cloth behind the knee to create space in the joint, or place a blanket under the hips to take pressure off the knees.

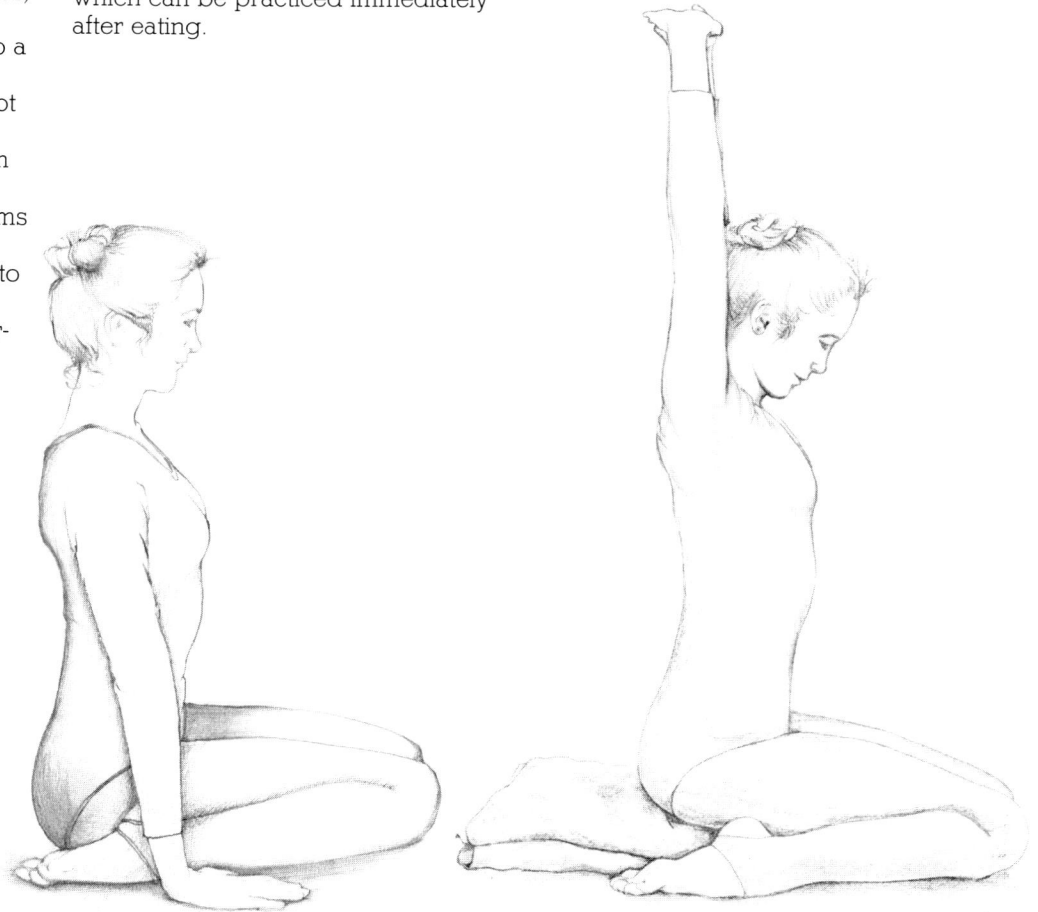

SQUATTING

Squat with the feet together flat on the floor, toes pointing straight ahead. If this is difficult, spread the feet a few inches apart. If the heels come off the floor place a blanket under the heels for support.

- press elbows against insides of knees, opening the thighs
- join palms in front of chest in *namaskar* (prayer) position
- inhale, press knees against elbows, and lift spine from pelvis
- hold for half a minute, and release on exhalation

Benefits
Squatting increases the flexibility of the ankles, stretches the front of the knees, and releases the hips. It aids digestion and elimination. Recommended for pregnant women, with feet wider apart.

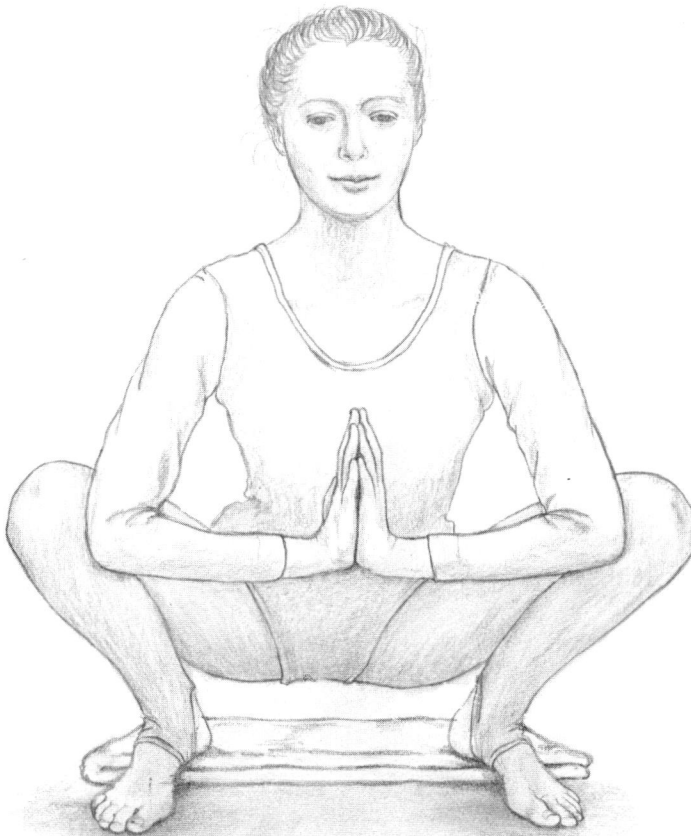

BADDHA KONASANA
(*baddha*, bound; *kona*, angle; bound angle pose)

Sit on the floor or against a wall with back erect and legs outstretched. Place a blanket under the sitting bones if the pelvis is tilting backwards.

- bend knees and draw heels close to torso
- press soles of feet together, holding feet or ankles with both hands, arms fully extended
- extend spinal column and lengthen inner thighs, so that knees descend towards floor
- hold for 2 or 3 minutes, breathing softly

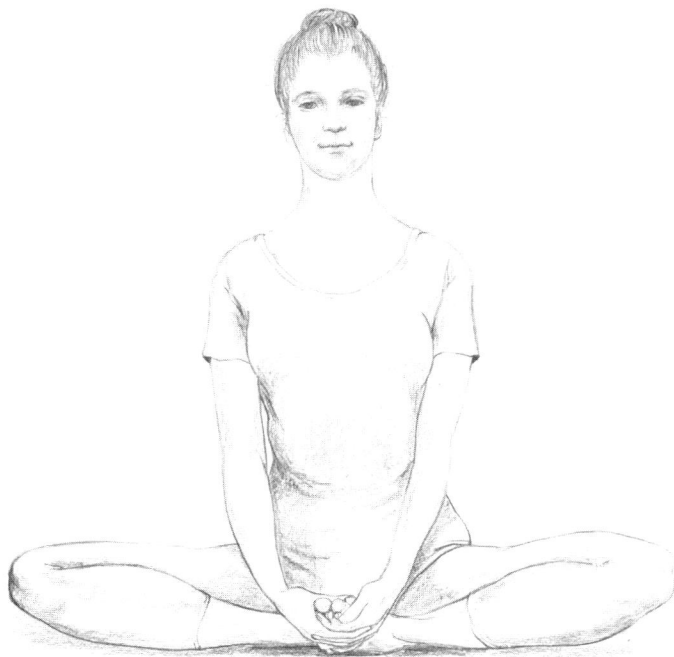

VARIATION
For this variation, you should sit with hips and upper back against a wall for support.

- place hands on upper thighs, and roll thighs out, to stretch groin area and open hips
- do not bounce knees or push them to floor — when inner thighs stretch, knees will descend naturally.

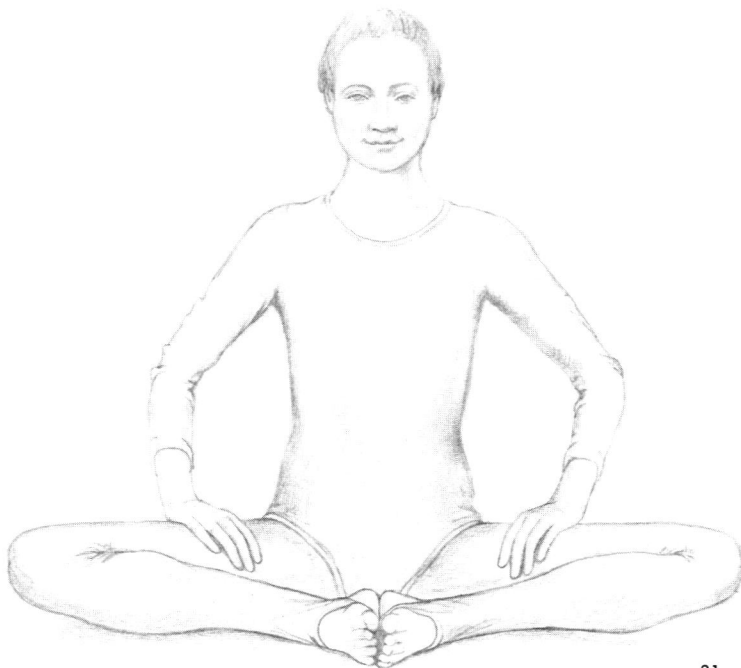

Benefits
Creates openness in the hips and flexibility in the knees; excellent as preparation for lotus and other meditation poses; also highly recommended for pregnant women.

Caution
If you experience pain in the knee, place a small rolled cloth behind the knee to create space in the joint. Do not practice this pose with persistent knee pain.

GOMUKHASANA

(go, cow; *mukha*, face; face of a cow pose)

Sit on the floor with legs outstretched and feet together.

- cross right leg *under* left leg, and bring right foot to left buttock
- cross left leg *over* right leg, and bring left foot to right buttock
- bring left knee directly over right knee
- raise right arm overhead, bend elbow, and place right hand between shoulders
- exhale, swing left arm behind back and catch hold of right hand — using a strap if necessary
- keep head erect and look straight ahead
- hold for half a minute, releasing tension in shoulders
- repeat to other side, changing cross of legs as well as arms

VARIATIONS

- sit on heels with knees together (*Vajrasana*) or sit between feet with knees together (*Virasana*)
- repeat arm movements as above

Benefits

Gomukhasana removes stiffness in the upper back, shoulder and neck. The cross-legged variation helps to relieve sciatic pain.

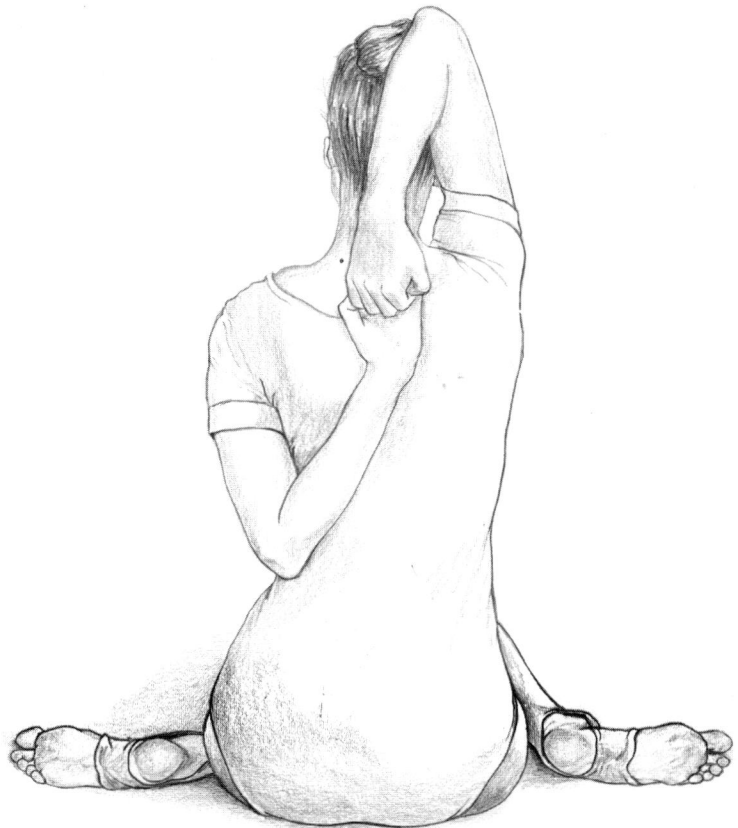

The asanas in this section are valuable for lengthening the back muscles, toning the spinal nerves, and massaging the abdominal organs. Initially, you may experience considerable resistance in forward bending because of tightness in the hamstring muscles at the back of the legs. These muscles will become flexible with consistent practice, and your whole range of movement will increase considerably. When the initial stiffness in the leg muscles is overcome, these forward bending postures have a very soothing effect on the nervous system and mind.

Before attempting any forward bending asanas, it is essential to understand the dynamics of performing the movement correctly, in order to avoid injury to the spine. In all forward bending postures, whether performed from a standing or sitting position, it is critical that the bending be done from the hip joints and not from the waist. As you begin to bend forward, extend the spine to its maximum, and tilt the pelvis so that the body folds at the hip joints and the front of the torso continues to lengthen.

Initially, if the back and hamstring muscles are very tight, you will not be able to bend forward very far. In this case, use a belt or strap around the feet to help you lift the pelvis and keep the spine extended. It will also help to sit at the edge of a folded blanket.

When the legs are extended, the knees should be kept straight, and the toes should point directly towards the ceiling. When the legs are bent, and there is pain in the knee, you can place a small rolled cloth behind the knee to create space in the joint. Do not continue to practice a posture with persistent knee pain.

Likewise students with a severe back injury, slipped disc or sciatica should practice sitting forward bends in a modified form — paying great attention to the straightness and lengthening of the spinal column.

JANUSHIRSHASANA
(*janu*, knees; *shirsha*, head; posture where head rests on knee)

Sit on the floor with legs outstretched and feet together. Place a folded blanket underneath the sitting bones.

- bend left knee, press calf to thigh, and place left thigh on floor
- extend left knee away from right leg, resting top of left foot on floor, with toes touching inner right thigh
- keep right leg active, with toes and knee pointing directly toward ceiling
- inhale, press left knee into floor, lift spinal column and turn center of chest to face center of right thigh
- exhale, bend forward from hip joints and take hold of right foot, using a strap if shoulders hunch or back is stiff
- inhale, stretch right leg and lengthen front of torso from pubic bone to chest, making back concave
- exhale, bring chest toward thigh, and lengthen back of head and neck toward feet
- keep arms fully extended — taking hold of wrist if hands reach beyond foot
- hold for half to one minute, releasing deeper into pose with each exhalation

Return to sitting position and repeat to other side.

Benefits
One of the most important poses, *Janushirshasana* prepares the beginner for more intense forward bends and develops the flexibility of hips and knees necessary for a good meditation posture.

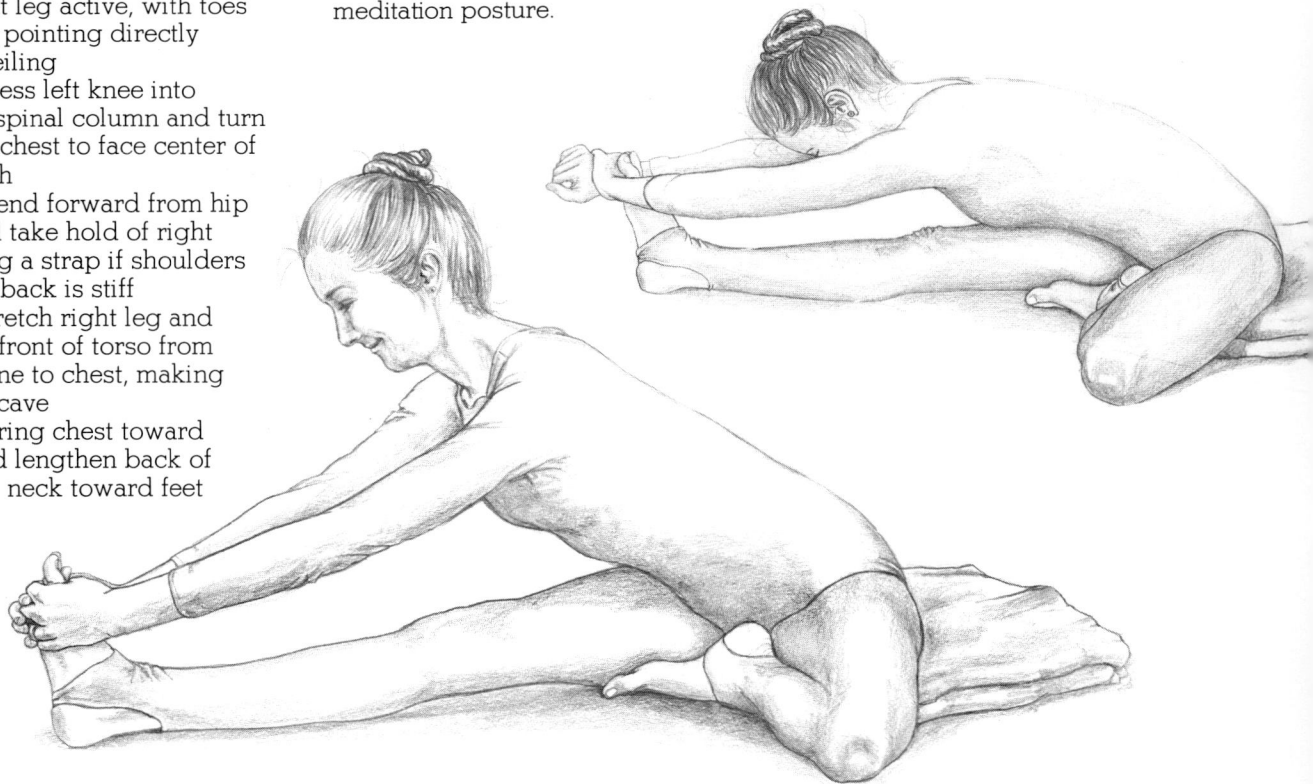

PREPARATION FOR HALF LOTUS

It is helpful to practice this preparation immediately before performing *Ardha Padma Paschimottanasana*, and before sitting in *Ardha Padmasana* or *Padmasana*.

Sit with the pelvis and back erect, and the legs outstretched.

- bend right knee and take hold underneath right ankle with both hands
- keep left leg straight, with knee and toes pointing directly to ceiling
- lift right foot as high as possible while keeping pelvis and spine erect
- make slow circular movements with foot, bringing foot as close to head as possible and down along torso
- repeat to other side
- do not reverse the movement: make circular motion only toward the body at the head and down along the torso.

Benefits
Creates openness in the hips and flexibility in the knees.

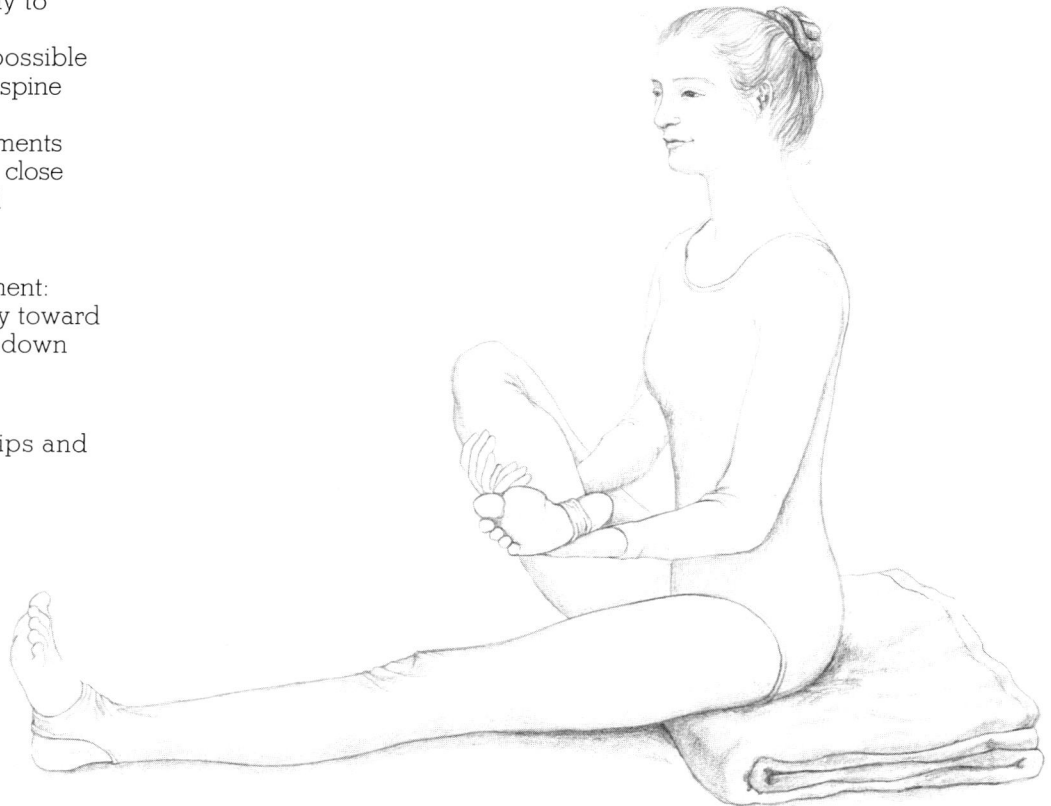

ARDHA PADMA PASCHIMOTTANASANA

(*ardha*, half; *padma*, lotus; *paschima*, west side or back; *uttan*, stretch; half-lotus back-stretching posture)

You will not be ready to practice this pose until the knee of the bent leg touches the floor in *Janushirshasana*. Sit on the floor with a blanket under the sitting bones, legs outstretched and heels together.

- bend right knee, place right foot on top of left thigh, with heel pressing into lower abdomen, as in half-lotus position
- keep left leg straight, with toes and knee pointing directly toward ceiling
- inhale, lift from base of spine and turn center of chest to face center of left thigh
- exhale, bend forward from hip joints, and take hold of left foot, using a strap if necessary
- keep arms fully extended — taking hold of wrist if hands reach beyond foot
- hold for half to one minute, releasing deeper into pose with each exhalation

Return to sitting position, and repeat to other side.

Benefits

In this pose, the heel massages the lower abdomen, and brings relief and stimulation to the intestines and abdominal organs.

Caution

If you experience pain in the knee, place a small rolled cloth behind the knee to create space in the joint. Do not practice this posture with persistent knee pain.

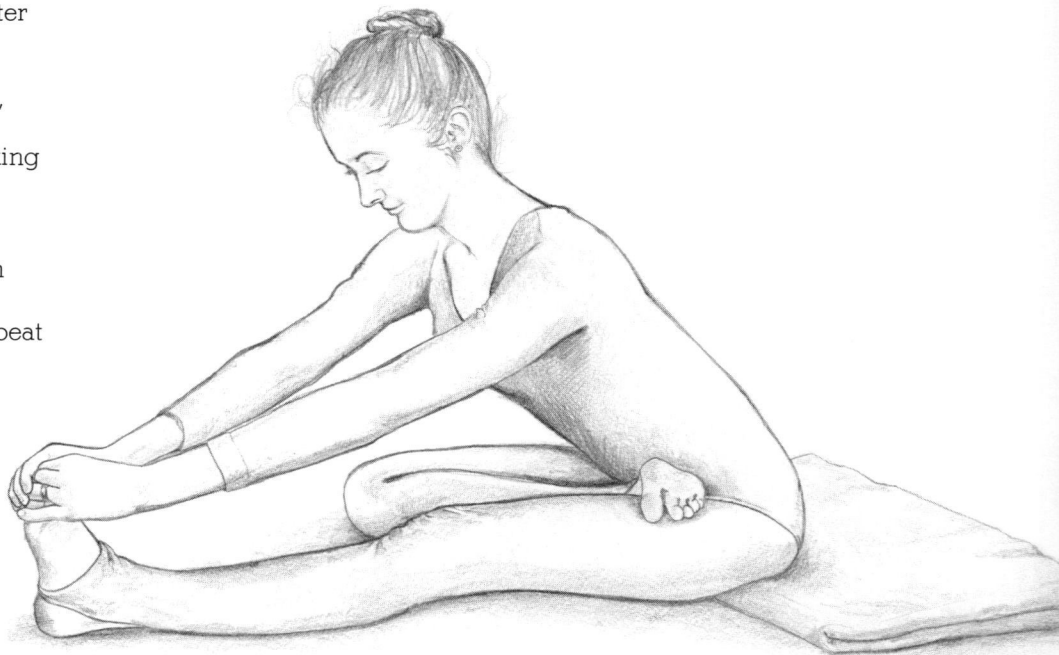

PASCHIMOTTANASANA

(*paschima*, west; *uttan*, stretch; posture that stretches west (back) side of body)

Sit on the floor with a blanket under the sitting bones, legs outstretched, and heels together.

VARIATION 1

For students with tight hamstrings and/or who suffer from lower back pain.

- place a strap around feet, with arms fully extended and shoulders drawn down
- keep legs straight with knees and toes pointing directly towards ceiling

- inhale, stretch legs and lift pelvis and spine vertically, so that vertebrae of lower back do not protrude
- hold for 1 or 2 minutes, breathing softly

VARIATION 2

For students who are more flexible in the hips and lower back.

- take hold of soles of feet, but do not let shoulders hunch
- keep legs straight with knees and toes pointing directly towards the ceiling
- inhale, stretch legs and lengthen front of torso from pubic bone to chest, making back concave
- exhale, bend forward from hip joints, bring chest toward thighs, and lengthen back of head and neck toward feet
- keep arms fully extended — taking hold of wrist if hands reach beyond feet

- hold for 1 to 5 minutes, releasing deeper into pose with each exhalation
- return to sitting position on inhalation

Benefits

This is one of the classic ancient postures referred to in the scriptures of Hatha Yoga: the *Hatha Yoga Pradipika, Gheranda Samhita,* and *Shiva Samhita.* In the *Hatha Yoga Pradipika,* the benefits of *Paschimottanasana* are described: "This foremost asana, *Paschimottan,* fans the fires of appetite, reduces obesity and cures all diseases of men." This forward bend is very soothing for the heart and for the nervous system. In addition, because of the contraction of the abdominal region, all organs are toned, particularly the liver, kidneys, pancreas and the female organs.

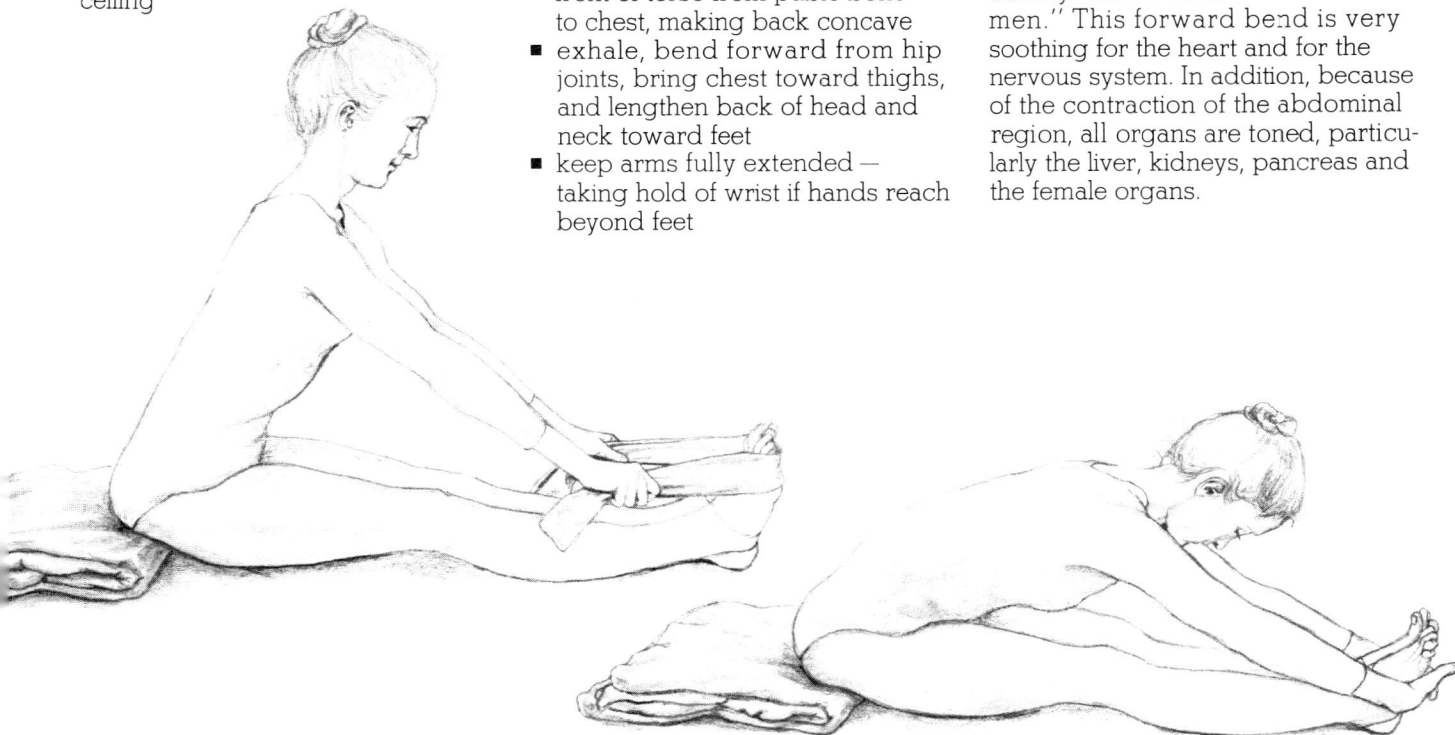

MANDUKASANA
(*manduka*, frog; frog pose)

This posture can be used for a brief relaxation between other postures.

Sit on your heels with the knees wide apart, so that the torso can rest between the thighs.

- exhale, bend forward from hips until forehead touches floor
- extend arms overhead, with palms down on floor, or fold arms and support forehead
- keep buttocks in contact with heels, and release lower back and abdomen
- hold for several minutes, or until you feel rested

Benefits
This pose is very relaxing and soothing to the nervous system. It is helpful for anyone with lower back problems and can also give relief from constipation.

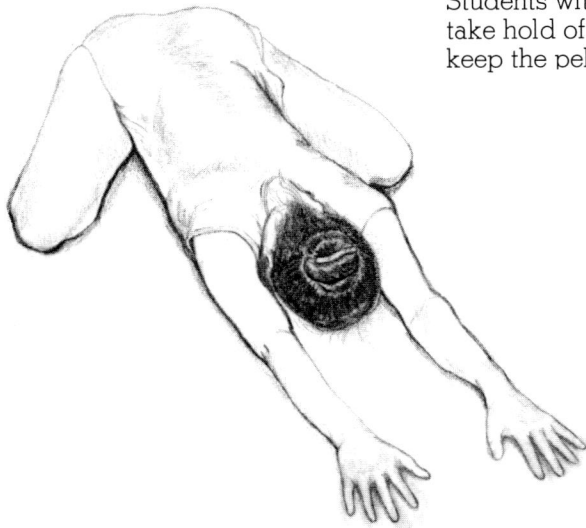

UPAVISTHA KONASANA
(*upavistha*, seated; *kona*, angle; seated angle pose)

Sit on the floor with a blanket under the sitting bones and back erect.

- spread legs as wide as possible without stressing inner knees
- inhale, press hands into floor to lift spine and make back concave
- exhale, bend forward from hip joints, lengthen torso from pubic bone to chest, and bring hands onto ankles, or onto floor directly ahead
- keep legs straight with knees and toes pointing toward ceiling throughout pose
- for more advanced students, release hips and lengthen front of body until torso rests on floor between legs
- hold for 1 or 2 minutes, breathing normally

Students with tight hamstrings should take hold of the feet with straps and keep the pelvis and back erect.

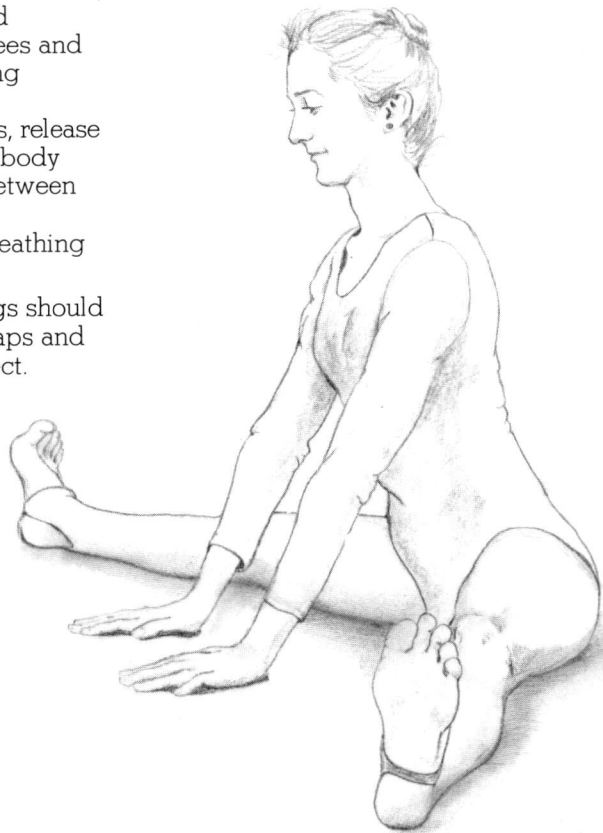

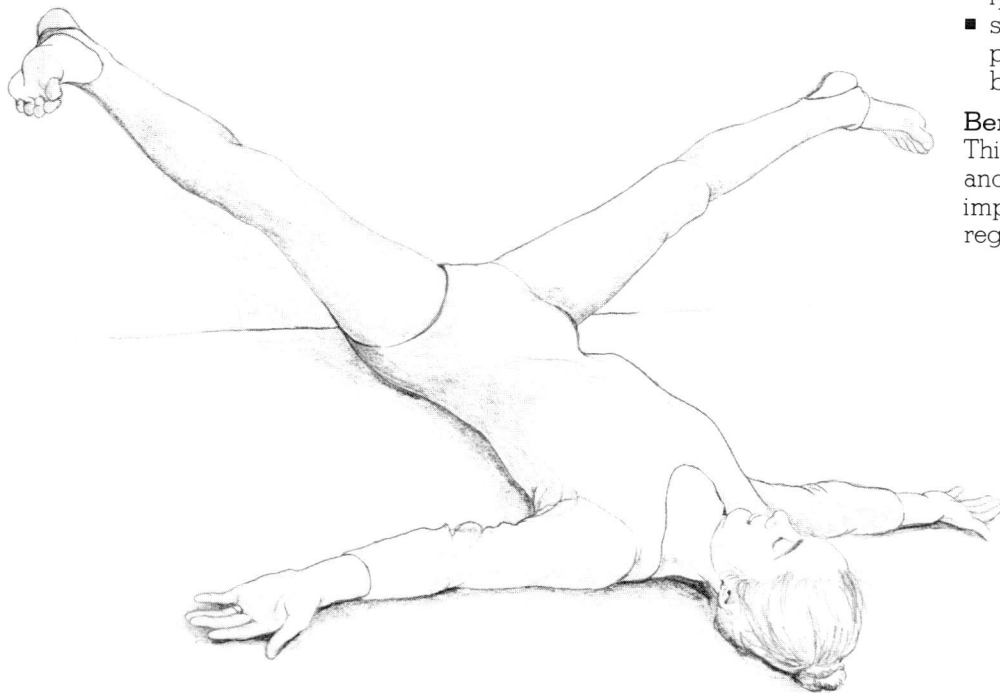

VARIATION 1

- lie against the wall with the legs stretched up the wall and the torso lying at 90° along the floor
- spread the legs apart as much as possible and relax the whole body breathing gently

Benefits

This pose stretches the inner thighs and opens the hips, and is especially important for women, as it helps to regulate the menstrual flow.

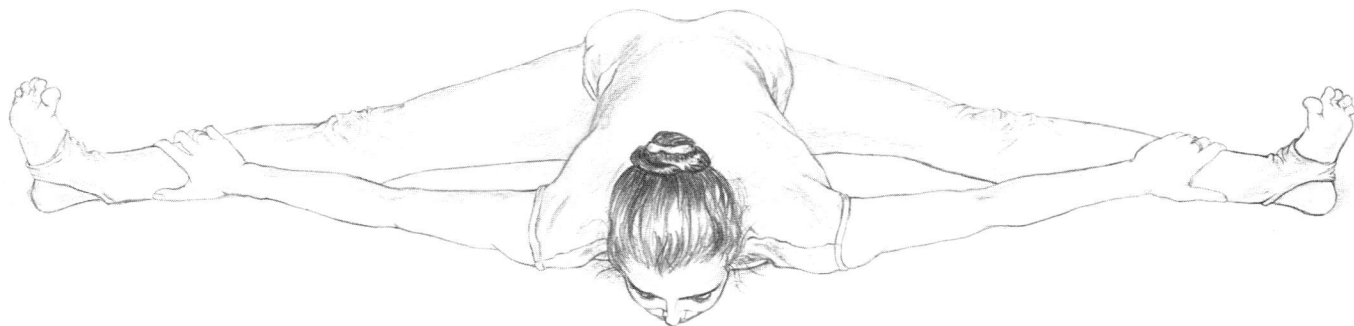

Backward Bending Postures

The asanas in this section bend the spinal column backwards, expand the chest and stretch the muscles along the front of the body. Backward bends are exhilarating and revitalizing due to their stimulating effect on the spinal nerves. The vertebrae and accompanying muscles and ligaments receive an additional supply of fresh blood, which rejuvenates the entire spine, maintaining its strength and flexibility. Also, the abdominal muscles and internal organs benefit greatly from being stretched and massaged.

When practicing back bends, it is important to maximize the opening of the upper back, and to keep the buttock muscles very firm. This will prevent painful compression of the lower back. If you have a spinal injury you should consult your doctor before undertaking the practice of these postures. While they can be beneficial for most people, they could aggravate an existing injury if practiced inappropriately.

SHALABHASANA
(*shalabha*, locust; locust pose)

Lie face down on a blanket, with arms extended along the sides. Bring the legs together, with feet touching, and toes pointed.

WARM-UP VARIATION
- exhale, raise right leg a few inches only, so that both hip bones stay in contact with floor
- keep right leg straight, contract buttocks, and stretch right thigh away from pelvis
- hold for half a minute, breathing softly, and release on exhalation
- realign body; repeat with other leg

COMPLETED POSE
- stretch arms back toward hips, with palms facing up
- inhale, lift chest, arms and legs off floor
- chest should be raised a few inches only, to arch upper back without causing strain or compression of lumbar
- keep arms parallel to floor, stretching from shoulders to fingers
- legs should be lifted a few inches only with knees straight and buttocks firm, extending back of thighs toward heels
- hold for half a minute, breathing softly, and release on exhalation

Benefits
Strengthens muscles of the thighs, buttocks and lumbar region, and thus helps to relieve lower back pain, especially for those suffering from slipped discs.

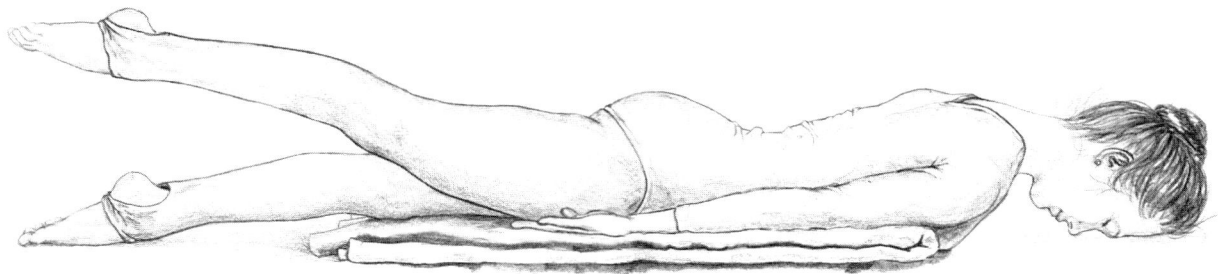

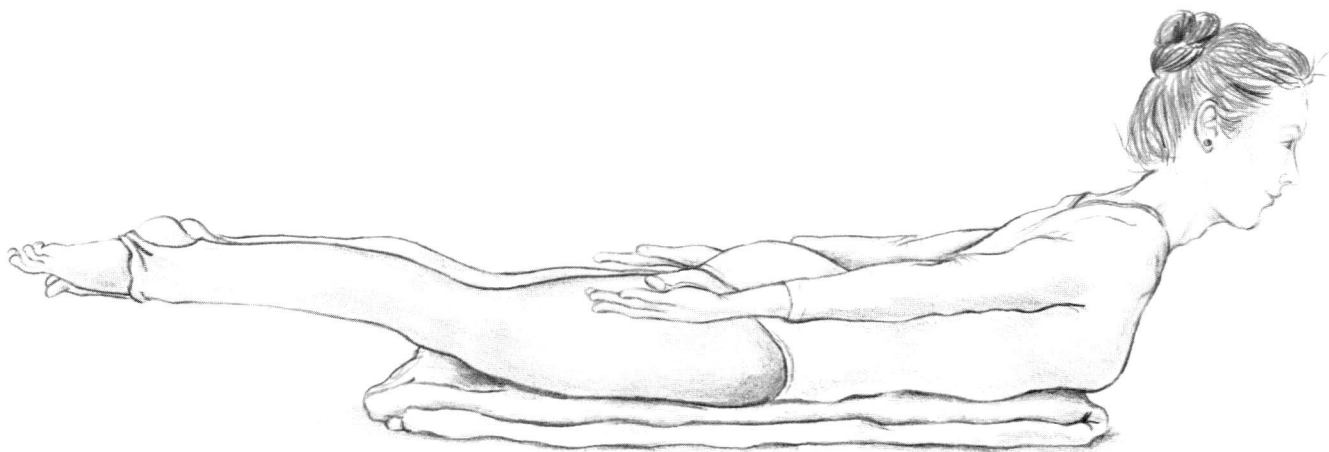

DHANURASANA
(*dhanu*, bow; bow posture)

Lie face down on a blanket, with the legs extended and feet together.

- exhale, bend legs toward buttocks, take hold of ankles and flex heels
- if grasping ankles with hands is difficult, try using a strap
- inhale, press tailbone towards floor and contract buttocks to protect lower back
- exhale, lift chest and thighs off floor, keeping knees and thighs parallel but not together
- press ankles away from head to create greater opening of upper back
- hold for a half a minute, and release on exhalation

Benefits
Opens upper chest and brings elasticity to the entire spine; massages abdominal organs, especially the liver and kidneys, thus relieving chronic constipation, poor digestion and liver sluggishness.

Caution
If you experience pain in the lower back in this pose, return to the practice of *Shalabhasana*, or seek advice from a teacher.

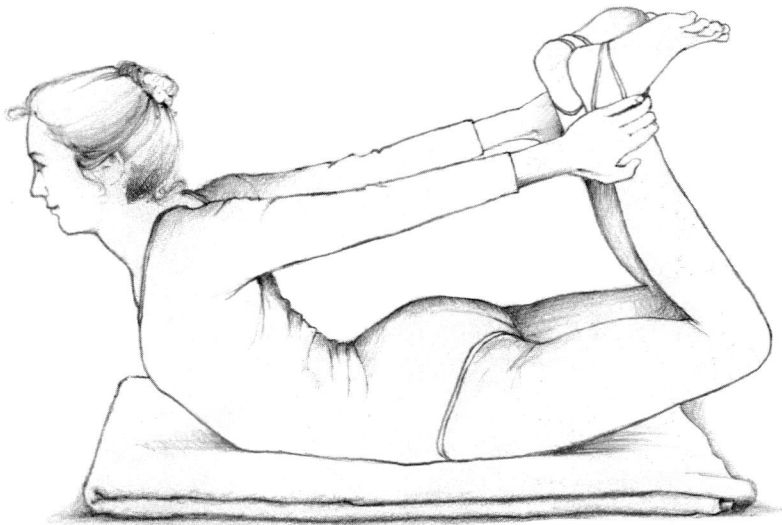

URDHVA MUKHA SVANASANA

(*urdhva*, upward; *mukha*, face; *svana*, dog; upward-facing dog)

Lie face down on the floor with legs extended back.

- move feet a few inches apart, parallel with hips, and curl toes under
- place hands with fingertips directly under shoulders and draw elbows back towards waist
- exhale, lift kneecaps, contract buttocks, and straighten arms to bring torso and legs off floor
- roll shoulders open to arch upper back, press arms down into floor, and lift spinal column
- keep buttocks firm, move tailbone deep into body, and stretch front thighs to protect lower back
- hold for half a minute, and release on exhalation

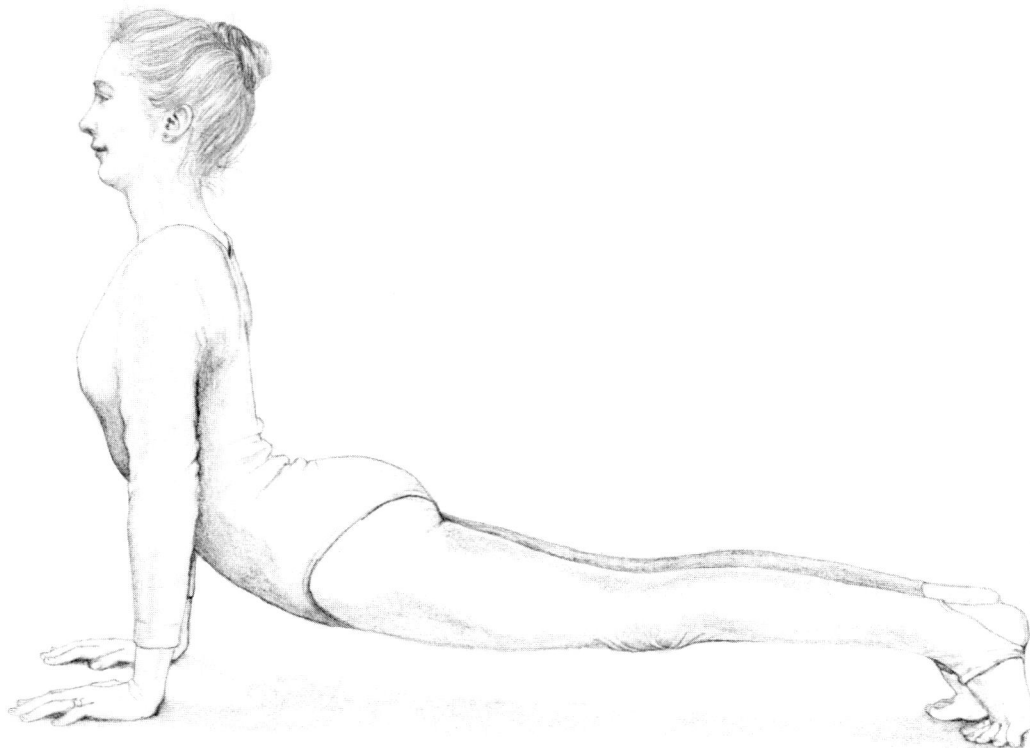

Benefits
Creates greater flexibility in the spine and improves circulation of the pelvic area, with less risk of lumbar compression when legs are actively lifting from floor.

Caution
If you experience back pain in this pose, try placing your hands on a low bench, platform or other raised surface. Even a rolled blanket will do. If pain persists, revert to easier backbends, and ask your teacher for advice.

Spinal Twist Postures

The spinal twist postures are especially valuable for opening the upper chest and shoulders, and for releasing any tension or discomfort of the spinal column. You will find it beneficial to follow backbends or intense forward bends with spinal twists, because of the relief they bring to the lower back. Regular practice of twisting postures stimulates the powerful spinal nerves, nourishes the discs, and strengthens and loosens the associated muscles of the back. The twisting movement also has a powerful influence on the abdominal organs, massaging them and bringing a fresh flow of blood to that area.

When practicing twists, it is important to lift the spinal column from the base with an inhalation. Then on exhalation, the twisting movement should begin from the pelvis and lower abdomen, not from the shoulders, so that the rib-cage remains free of strain and tension, and the spinal energy moves upwards.

BHARADVAJASANA
(dedicated to the sage *Bharadvaja*)

Sit on the floor with legs outstretched and a blanket under the sitting bones to keep the hips level.

- draw left leg back to side of hip, with top of left foot on floor
- place right foot on top of left thigh as in half-lotus — or if knees and hips are stiff, place right foot on floor touching inner left thigh
- place left hand on right knee, swing right arm behind back on exhalation, and take hold of right foot — or use a strap to hold foot if necessary
- inhale, lift from base of spine, and press sitting bones to floor
- exhale, twist torso to right, and turn head to look over right shoulder
- hold pose for half a minute, breathing normally
- release, and repeat to other side

Benefits
This simple twist makes the spinal column more supple and opens the shoulders. It is very beneficial for those with stiff backs or arthritis.

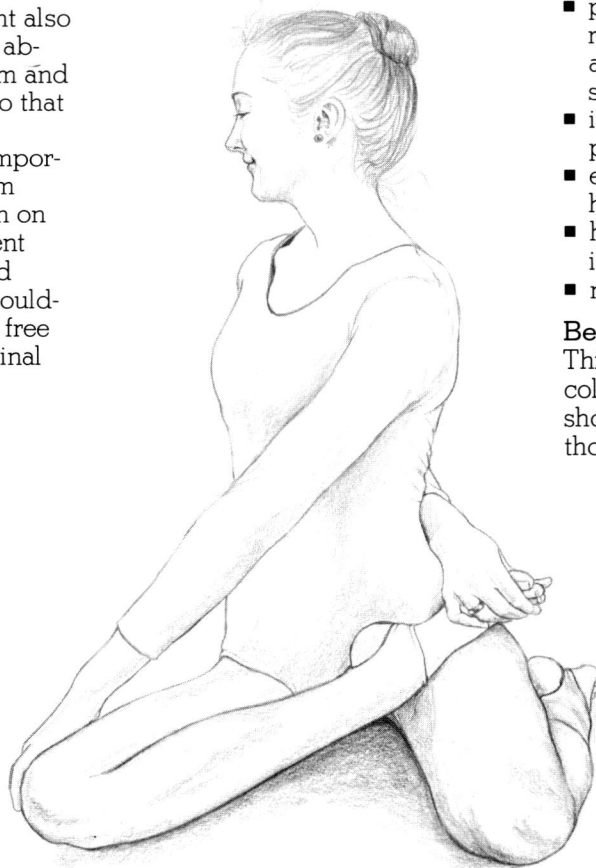

MARICHYASANA
(dedicated to the great sage *Marichi*)

In this pose, twist *away* from the bent leg.

VARIATION 1
Sit on the floor with legs outstretched and a blanket under the hips.

- bend left knee and bring heel in close to buttocks
- turn torso to right, and press upper left arm against left knee
- bring left ribcage to meet left thigh, and wrap left arm around outside of left leg
- take right arm behind back and clasp hands or wrist — or use a strap if you cannot catch hands
- lift spinal column, deepen twist, and turn head over right shoulder
- hold pose for half a minute, and repeat to other side.

Benefits
As for *Bharadvajasana*.

In next two variations of this pose, twist *towards* the bent knee.

VARIATION 2
Sit at the edge of a blanket with legs outstretched and feet together.

- bend left knee, drawing heel close to left buttock
- place left hand on floor behind hips, lean weight onto hand, and turn chest and abdomen beyond left thigh
- pause for several breaths to allow body to accept new position
- bend right arm, bringing upper arm in front of left knee, and turn torso even more by lifting from base of spine
- bring right armpit in contact with left knee, so that ribcage touches thigh
- keep right leg outstretched with kneecap lifted and toes pointing directly towards ceiling
- hold for half a minute, breathing normally and opening the chest

Repeat to the other side.

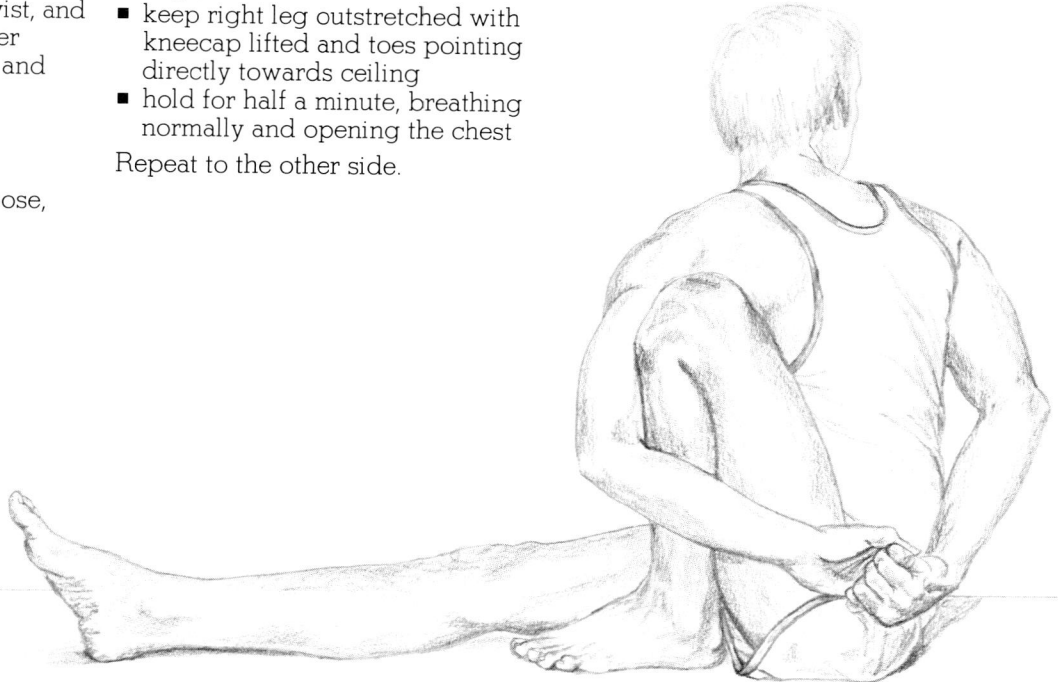

VARIATION 3

If the ribcage comes in contact with the thigh, repeat the pose with the following additions:

- twist right arm around left knee, and place hand at back of waist
- exhale, swing left arm behind back, clasping left wrist with right hand — or use a strap if hands do not meet
- keep right leg fully extended, and lift from base of spine
- head may turn either towards or away from extended leg
- hold for half a minute, breathing softly, and release on exhalation

Repeat to the other side.

Benefits

This twisting posture releases the vertebrae, tones the spinal nerves, and makes the back muscles supple. It massages the abdominal organs and the intestines, thereby relieving digestive ailments.

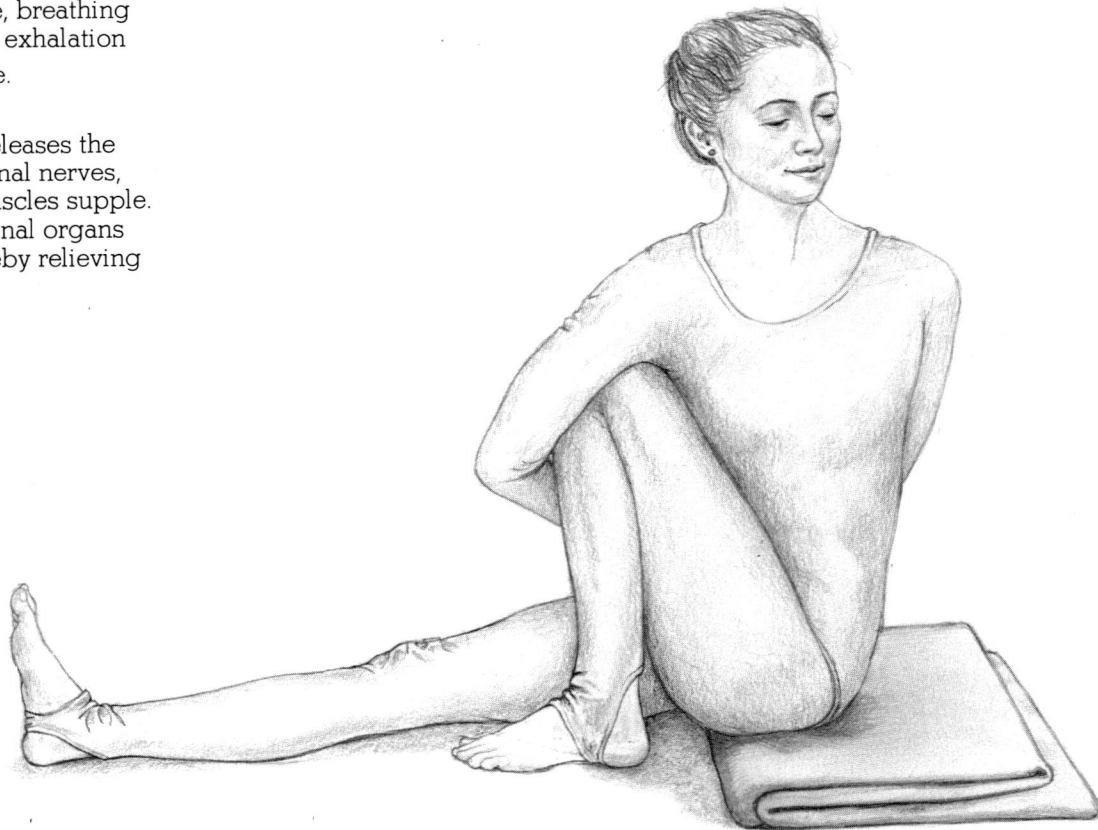

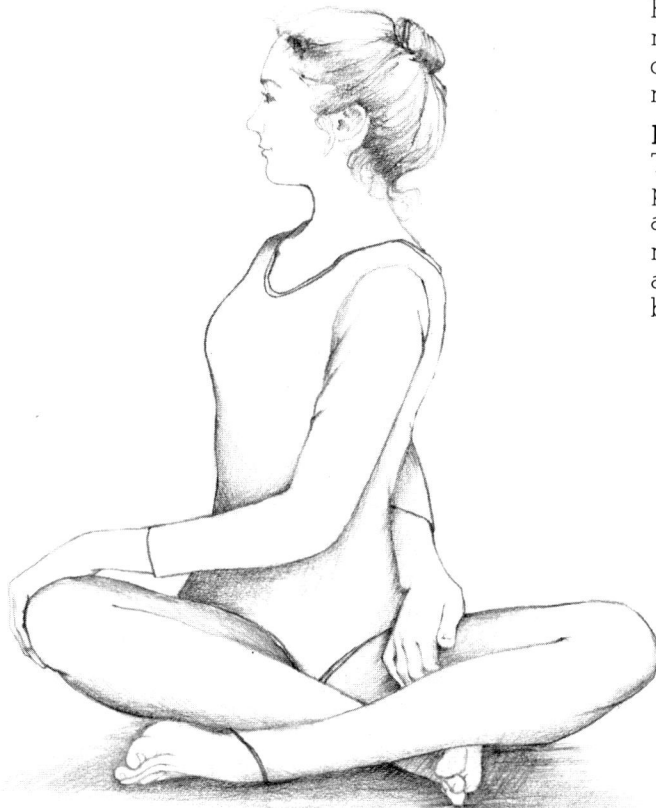

CROSS-LEGGED TWIST

Sit in a cross-legged position.

- place left hand on right knee and right hand behind back
- inhale, lift spinal column
- exhale, gently pull on knee, twist upper body toward right and look over right shoulder
- check that crown of head remains directly over tailbone
- inhale, return to front
- reverse hand positions and twist in opposite direction

Repeat two or three times, letting the movement flow with the breath. Then change the cross of the legs, and repeat an equal number of times.

Benefits

This gentle twisting movement can be practiced in any cross-legged position, and is helpful both before and after meditation for lubricating the spine and reducing stiffness in the lower back.

Shoulderstand Series

Swami Muktananda described *Sarvangasana* (shoulderstand) as one of the most valuable asanas. He often prescribed its practice as a panacea for many physical ailments, and recommended it rather than the head-stand for meditators. Not only does *Sarvangasana* have a direct effect on the thyroid and parathyroid glands, which regulate metabolism, but it also soothes the nerves, calms the mind, and brings a sense of harmony and inner balance.

The asanas in this chapter should be practiced together in the sequence given. These postures release tightness of the neck and shoulders and develop the strength of the back, essential for a comfortable and steady meditation posture.

SETU BANDHASANA
(*setu bandha*, construction of a bridge; bridge pose)

This pose can be practiced before *Sarvangasana* (shoulderstand) to open the upper chest and release the shoulder joints and/or after *Sarvanga-sana* to release tension in the lower back.

Lie on your back with the shoulders at the smooth edge of a folded blanket, leaving a space between the neck and floor.

- bend knees, and place feet several inches apart but close to buttocks
- keep feet and thighs parallel throughout pose — knees should press towards one another, not drop away
- exhale, press heels into floor, and lift pelvis towards ceiling
- contract buttocks and extend thighs toward knees to lengthen lower back
- roll upper arms out, and come high onto shoulders
- hands can be placed on upper back, as for shoulderstand — on buttocks, for support of hips — or on ankles, for leverage in lifting chest
- hold for half a minute, breathing normally
- exhale, and roll down slowly from upper back, releasing one vertebrae at a time

Benefits
This is a mild and therapeutic back-bend, which helps to relieve pain in the sacroiliac joint, or tension in the neck and shoulders caused by a rounded back.

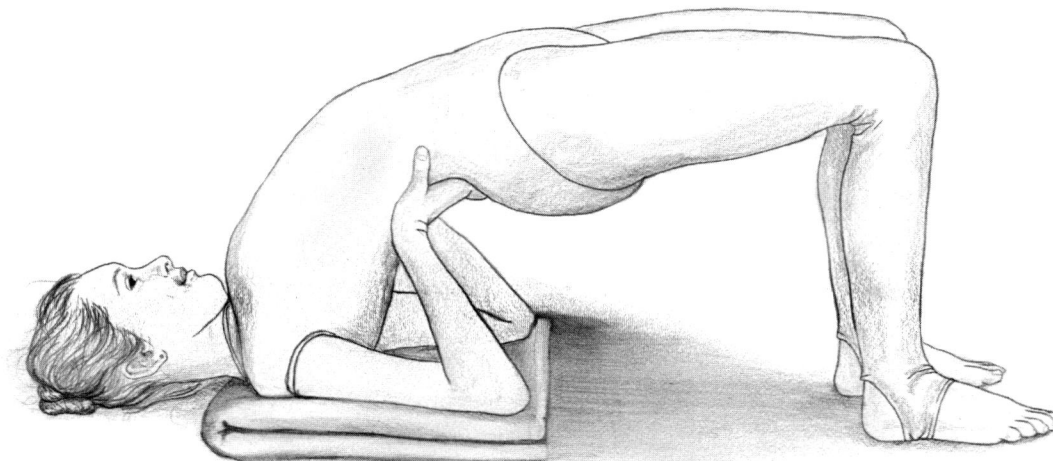

SARVANGASANA

(*sarva*, all; *arga*, limbs; posture for the whole body)

In *Sarvangasana* the weight of the body should balance on the shoulders and arms, not the neck, as continued pressure on the neck will destroy the natural cervical curve. You can avoid damage to the neck by using a thick blanket under the shoulders and upper back, with the head resting on the floor. Fold the blanket wide enough so that it will fit under your shoulders and elbows.

Lie on your back with your shoulders at the smooth edge of a folded blanket, legs outstretched, and arms by your sides with palms down.

- roll shoulders back and open chest
- exhale, press hands into floor, bend knees into chest, and lift pelvis toward ceiling
- bend elbows, press upper arms down to lift shoulder blades off floor, and come as high on shoulders as possible
- place hands on back close to shoulder blades with palms flat if possible
- bring elbows in so that upper arms are parallel — using a strap if necessary
- lift thighs toward ceiling, straighten legs, and keep ankles together, with soles of feet parallel to ceiling
- firm buttocks and thighs, draw tailbone deep into body, and stretch inner thighs toward ceiling

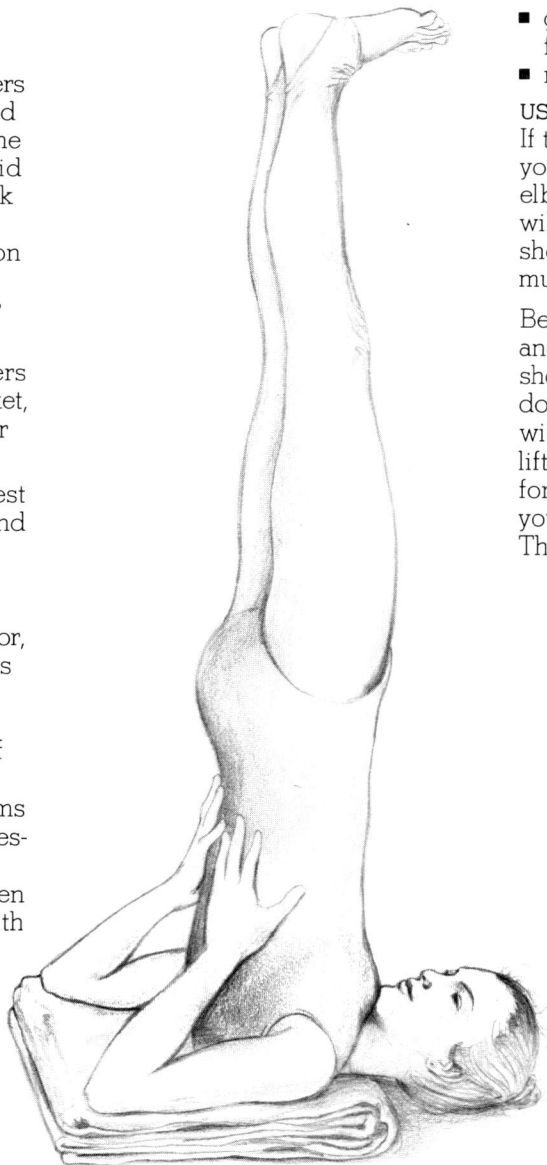

- let ribcage rest on hands, soften eyes, and relax neck and throat
- gradually increase time of holding from 1 to 10 minutes
- move directly into *Halasana*

USE OF STRAP

If the elbows slide out to the side, you can tie a strap just above the elbows to keep them in place. This will help you to lift higher onto the shoulders, and will make the pose much easier to hold.

Begin by folding your strap in half, and measuring the width of your shoulders. Tie the strap before lying down, and place it by your side within easy reach. When you have lifted the pelvis off the floor, reach for the strap and place it around your arms, just above the elbows. Then ascend into the full pose.

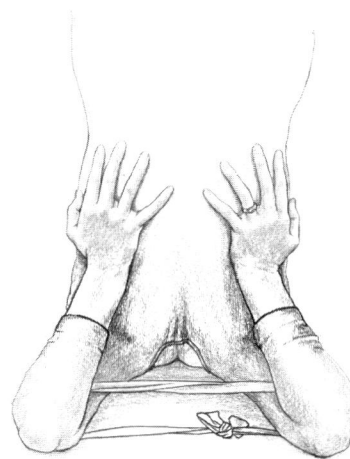

SARVANGASANA (Modified)

Some people find it difficult to lift the body perpendicular to the floor, due to inflexibility of the spine, tight shoulders, or a neck injury. In such cases, the following variation of the shoulderstand can be used.

Lie on your back with buttocks touching the base of a wall, and legs extended up the wall. Make sure that your blanket is placed evenly under the shoulders and that your neck is free.

- bend knees, place soles of feet on wall, and lift pelvis to vertical position
- roll shoulders under, and bring elbows in so that upper arms are parallel
- place hands as high on upper back as possible, and let ribcage rest on hands
- firm buttocks and thighs, press tailbone deep into body, and lengthen inner thighs towards knees
- soften eyes, and relax neck, throat, and upper chest
- hold for 1 to 3 minutes, breathing softly
- then lower pelvis by rounding upper back, and come down one vertebra at a time

When this posture becomes easier, you can try extending the legs up the wall, with knees straight and heels only resting on the wall. Then for brief intervals you can bring the legs away from the wall.

Benefits

In the inverted position the blood flow is reversed and easily recirculated through the heart. This is beneficial for varicose veins, constipation and respiratory ailments. The vital organs receive a fresh supply of blood, and the heart rests. *Sarvangasana* is also very soothing to the nervous system, and, if practiced before retiring, it can help eliminate tension and promote restful sleep.

Caution

Those with high blood pressure should not do *Sarvangasana*. They can practice *Halasana*, however, increasing the time very gradually. Women should not do *Sarvangasana* or other inverted poses during menstruation. Do not practice *Sarvangasana* with persistent neck pain, pressure in the eyes, or tension headaches, but seek advice from a competent teacher.

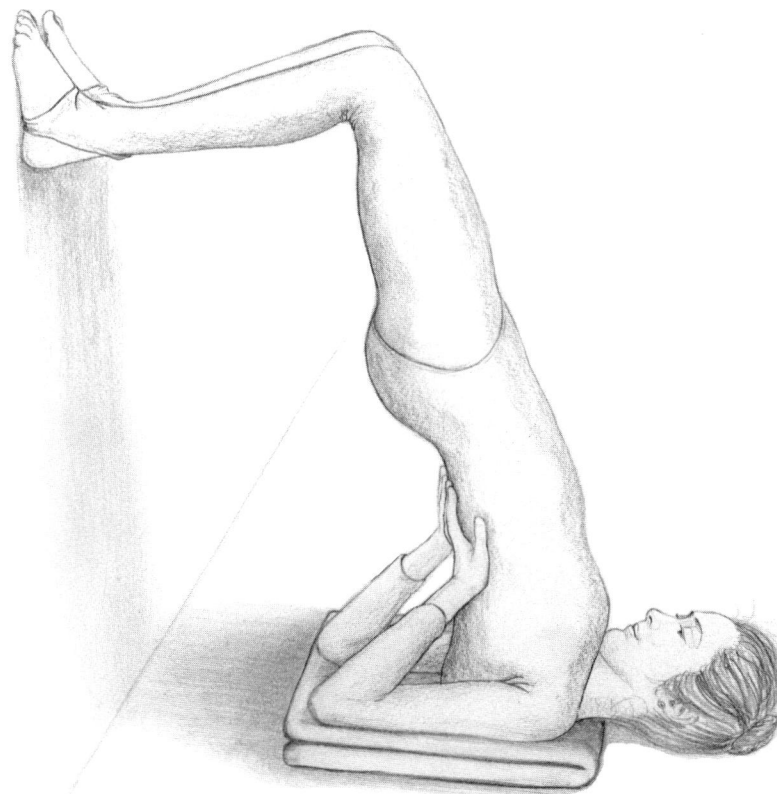

HALASANA
(*hala*, plow; plow posture)

Practice *Halasana*, immediately after *Sarvangasana* (shoulderstand), using a folded blanket under the shoulders to avoid strain on the neck.

From *Sarvangasana*

- lower legs slowly overhead, until toes touch floor, keeping knees straight and legs fully extended
- if lower back and hamstrings are tight, bring feet to rest on a chair, bench or other elevated surface
- keep hands on back as for *Sarvangasana*, or extend arms away from head pressing palms into floor
- press upper arms down to lift shoulder blades off floor, and come as high on shoulders as possible
- lengthen inner thighs and lift pelvis toward ceiling, so that spine is fully extended
- soften eyes, and relax neck and throat
- gradually increase time of holding from 1 to 5 minutes
- to release, place hands on floor and roll down slowly

Benefits
Same as for *Sarvangasana*. In addition, the abdominal organs receive a beneficial massage, which stimulates digestion. *Halasana* is especially good for those with high blood pressure, but the feet should rest on an elevated surface, not on the floor.

Caution
If pain occurs in the lower back, use a chair, bench or other support under the feet. If pain persists, seek advice from a competent teacher.

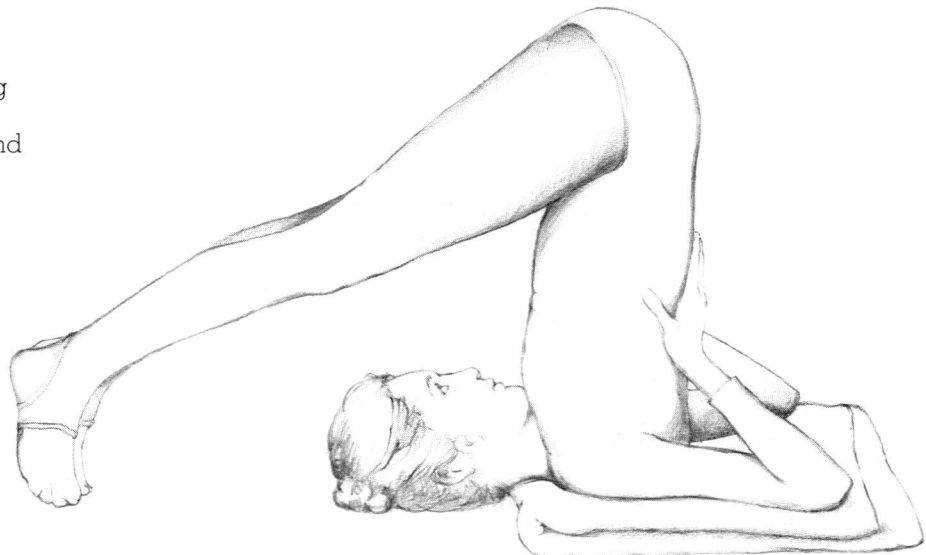

KARNIPIDASANA

(*karna*, ears; *pida*, pressure; ear-pressing posture)

This posture can be performed in sequence after *Sarvangasana* and *Halasana*.

From *Halasana* (plow pose)

- bend knees, and draw thighs toward chest, so that knees are next to ears and against shoulders
- extend arms away from head, interlock fingers and press upper arms into floor to come high onto shoulders
- then place hands on back as for *Sarvangasana* or bring arms overhead and take hold of feet
- hold position for half a minute, breathing normally
- to release, place hands on floor and roll down slowly

Benefits
This posture stretches the entire back, particularly the upper back, and increases circulation in the spine. It also massages the abdominal organs.

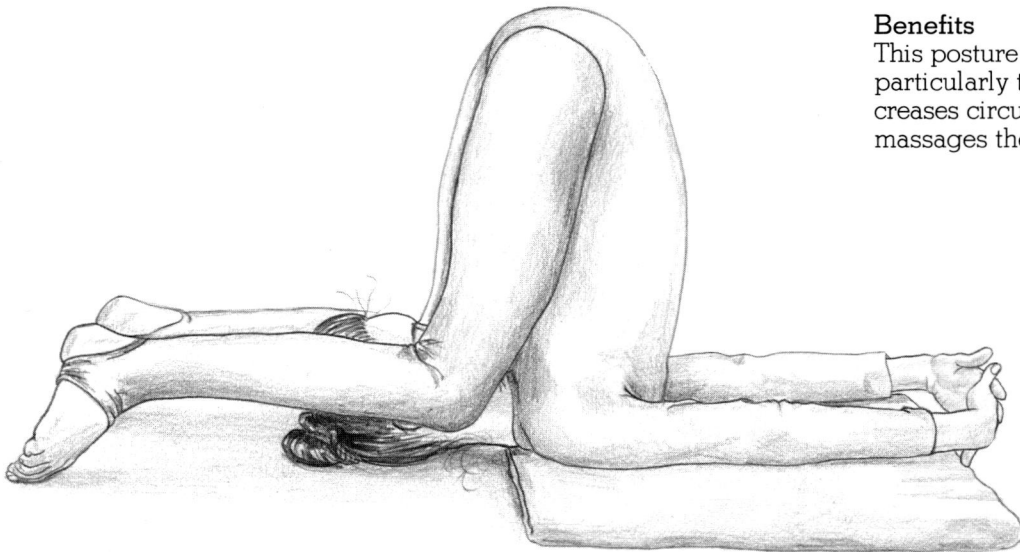

PAVANA MUKTASANA

(*pavana*, wind; *mukta*, to release, wind-releasing pose)

The shoulderstand sequence should be followed by one or two counterposes which stretch the lower back and release the neck. *Pavana Muktasana* can be practiced for this purpose, as can any of the following poses: *Setu Bandhasana; Jatara Parivartanasana; Supta Padangusthasana.*

Lie on your back with legs extended.

- exhale, draw knees to chest
- press thighs firmly to chest, with arms clasped around legs
- breathe softly, release tension of abdomen, and allow lower back to lengthen
- exhale, lift forehead to knees, hold for several seconds, and return head and shoulders to floor on inhalation

VARIATION
- increase stretch by interlacing fingers behind balls of feet
- lift head to knees on exhalation, and release on inhalation

Benefits

This position is prescribed for relieving intestinal gas and constipation. It stretches and loosens the lower back, and massages the abdominal organs.

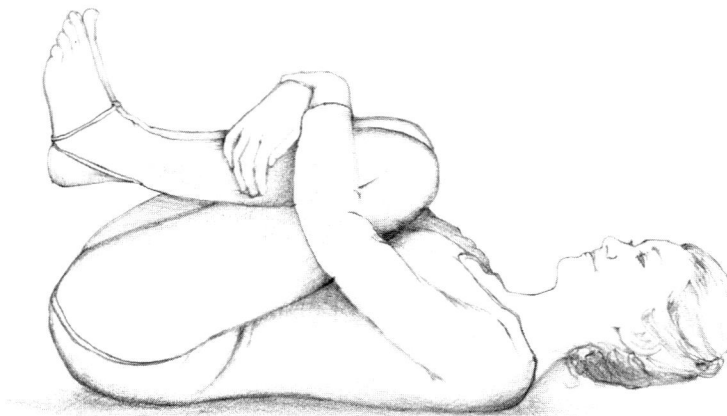

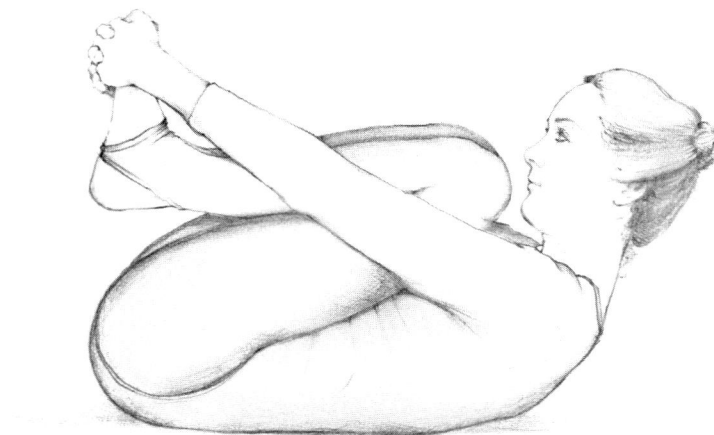

Reclining Postures

The postures in this chapter are primarily concerned with the abdomen and lower back. When the abdominal wall is weak, there is no adequate support for the lower back; the pelvis tilts forward in an exaggerated manner, the lumbar spine becomes overarched, and back strain results. The reclining postures help to reverse this process by strengthening the abdominal muscles.

These postures also give considerable relief from lower back discomfort by lengthening the back muscles, releasing the hip joints and realigning the pelvis. Because the reclining poses provide such direct relief for lower back problems, it is recommended that you perform them towards the end of your daily practice, in order to remove any aches or tensions created by intense forward bends, backward bends, or shoulderstand.

UTTANA PADASANA I
(*uttana*, upright; *pada*, foot; leg-lifting posture)

Lie on your back with legs together and arms by the sides. Place hands under buttocks, with palms down, or put a blanket under body from tailbone to thighs, to give support to lower back.

- keep left leg straight, with knee and toes pointing directly toward ceiling
- bend right knee and draw knee to chest, then straighten leg to vertical position and lower almost to floor
- repeat this cycling movement several times without letting heel touch floor
- then repeat with other leg
- now reverse direction of cycling movement, by raising right leg vertically, bending knee to chest, and then extending leg just above floor level
- repeat reverse cycling movement several times without letting heel touch floor
- repeat with other leg

Benefits
In addition to strengthening the back and abdominal muscles these cycling movements tone the abdominal organs, improving digestion and elimination. They are particularly beneficial for women whose abdomens are weak from childbirth.

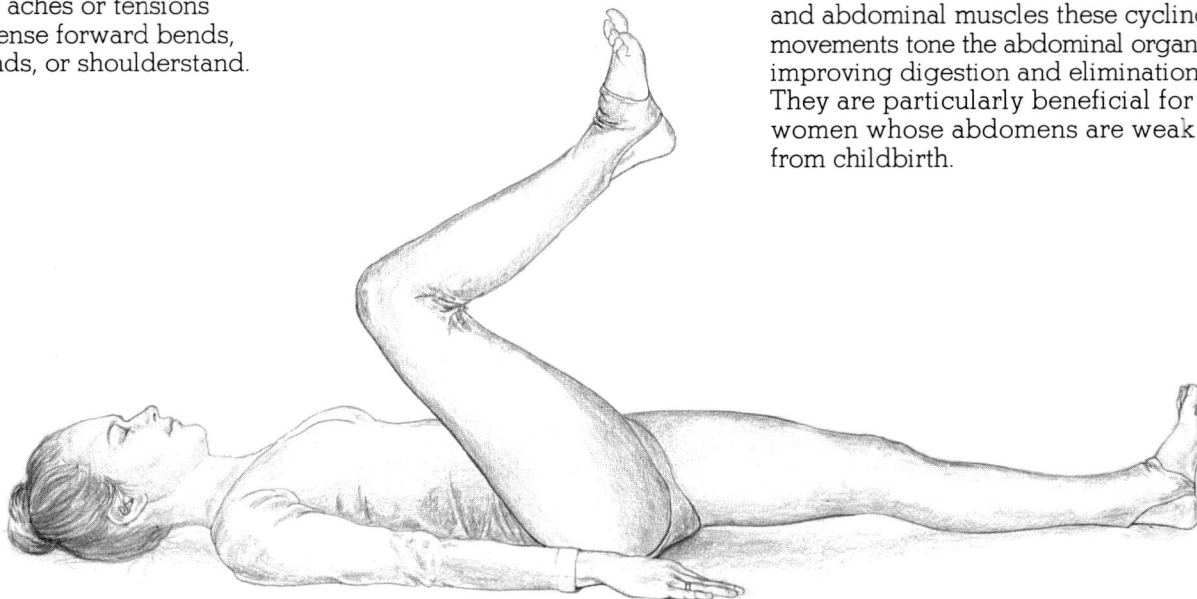

UTTANA PADASANA II

Lie on your back with legs together and arms by the sides. If you have a weak lower back, place a folded blanket under the sitting bones and thighs. This will prevent the pelvis from tilting forward when you raise your legs and thus protect the lower back from stress.

- inhale, press palms and lower back to floor
- exhale, raise legs to 90° angle
- inhale, keep legs fully extended and kneecaps lifted
- exhale, gradually lower legs to 60° angle, and hold for a few seconds breathing normally
- exhale, lower legs till only 2 or 3 inches from floor, firming buttocks and lengthening inner thighs
- release on exhalation

Repeat several times.

VARIATION
When the lower back has been strengthened, you can do this pose with arms stretched overhead on floor.

Benefits
Strengthens the back and abdominal muscles.

Caution
If you feel back strain during this pose, bend the knees and come down immediately. This posture should not be attempted by those with back injuries or by pregnant women.

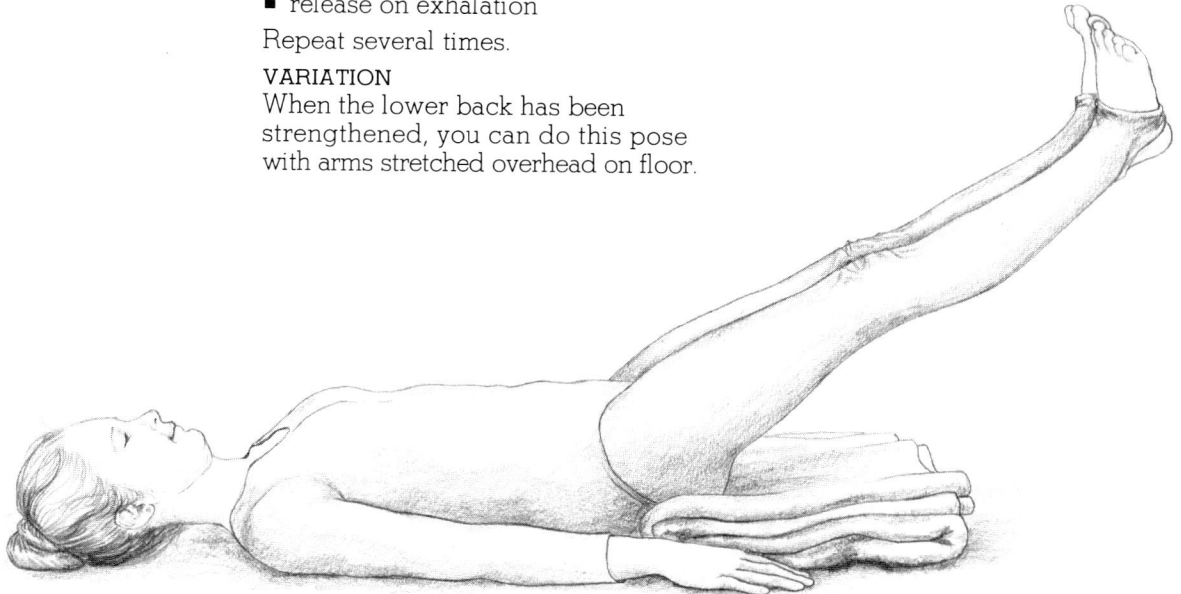

JATHARA PARIVARTANASANA
(*jathara*, stomach; *parivartana*, turning; stomach-turning posture)

VARIATION 1
Lie on your back with legs together and arms extended out to the side at shoulder level, with palms facing down.

- place arch of right foot on top of left knee
- exhale and twist pelvis to left, bringing right knee towards floor
- turn head to right and extend right arm out from center of back, bringing right shoulder in contact with floor.
- extend left thigh toward heel, and allow abdominal muscles to stretch
- hold for half a minute, breathing normally

VARIATION 2
Lie on your back with legs together and arms extended out to the side at shoulder level, palms facing down.

- inhale, lengthen lower back toward heels
- exhale, raise legs to vertical position, keeping knees straight and feet together

- maintain this position for several breaths
- exhale, lower legs toward left hand, pressing ankle bones together
- beginners can let legs rest on floor — more advanced students can hold feet a few inches off floor to strengthen abdomen
- turn head to right and extend right arm from center of back, bringing right shoulder closer to floor

- draw abdominal muscles to the right
- hold for a few breaths, and raise legs on exhalation

Repeat to the other side, and then slowly lower legs to starting position on exhalation.

Benefits
The gentle twisting action helps to relieve discomfort of the lower back. All the abdominal organs are toned, and excess weight around the hips is reduced.

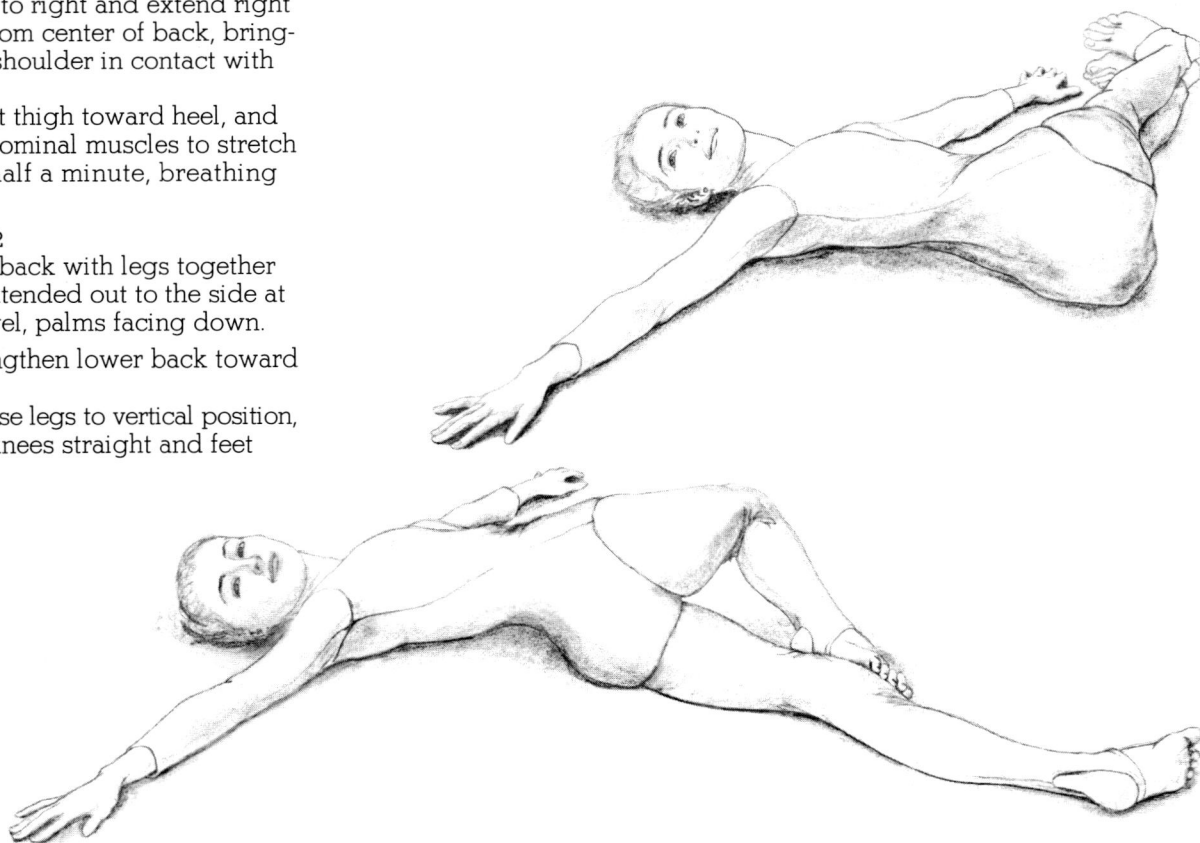

SUPTA PADANGUSTHASANA

(*supta*, lying down; *pada*, foot; *angustha*, big toe; reclining toe-holding pose)

VARIATION 1

In this variation, it is important to keep the raised leg straight, so that the hamstrings receive maximum stretch.

Lie on your back with legs together and arms by the side.

- inhale, raise right leg perpendicular to floor
- take hold of right big toe with right hand, and press left palm onto left thigh
- if hamstrings are tight, hold onto right foot with a strap, and bring leg to position where it can straighten
- keep left leg fully extended along floor, with knee and toes pointing directly towards ceiling
- inhale, lengthen back of right thigh towards heel
- exhale, release tension in abdomen and hips, and gradually draw leg closer to chest
- hold for up to one minute, breathing softly

Repeat to the other side.

VARIATION 2

Lie on your back with legs together and arms by the side.

- inhale, raise right leg perpendicular to floor
- exhale, bend right knee towards chest
- take hold of right foot with both hands, or with a strap if arms cannot reach foot comfortably
- inhale, stretch left leg towards heel, with knee and toes pointing directly towards ceiling
- exhale, press right knee towards armpit, bringing foot directly above knee to form a 90° angle at knee joint
- if knee comes easily to armpit, move right leg slightly to side, and press right knee gradually towards floor
- hold for 1 to 2 minutes, breathing softly Repeat to the other side.

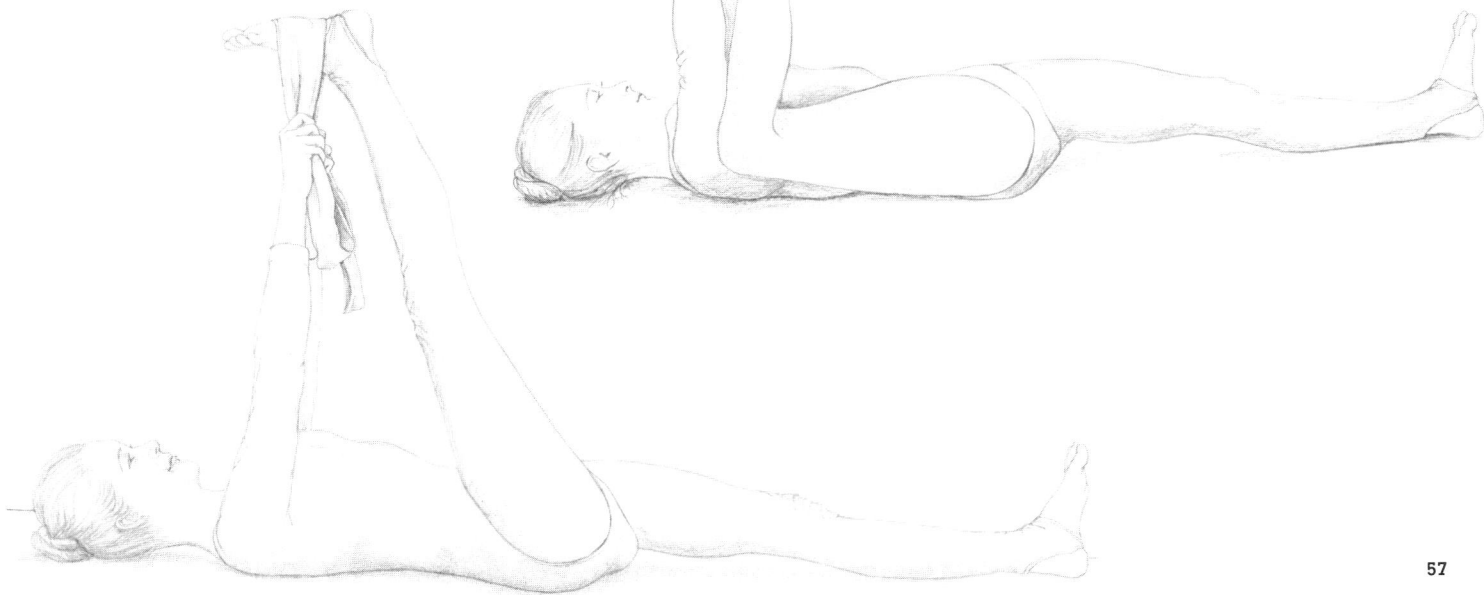

VARIATION 3

In this variation, it is important to keep the raised leg straight, so that the inner thigh receives optimum stretch. Lie on your back with legs extended and arms by the side, parallel to the wall and about two feet away.

- inhale, raise left leg vertically, keeping kneecap lifted
- exhale, lower left foot onto wall rotate left thigh out and draw left foot towards shoulder level
- if stretch of inner left thigh is too intense, or if you feel a pull at inner knee, move body nearer to wall, and left foot higher up wall
- if you feel no stretch of inner left thigh, move body further from wall, so that left foot comes nearer to floor, and inner left thigh receives a gentle stretch
- keep right leg fully extended along floor, with knee and toes pointing directly towards ceiling
- hold for 1 to 2 minutes, breathing softly

Benefits

All variations of this pose stretch the hamstrings, create mobility in the hips, and relieve discomfort from sciatica and other lower back problems.

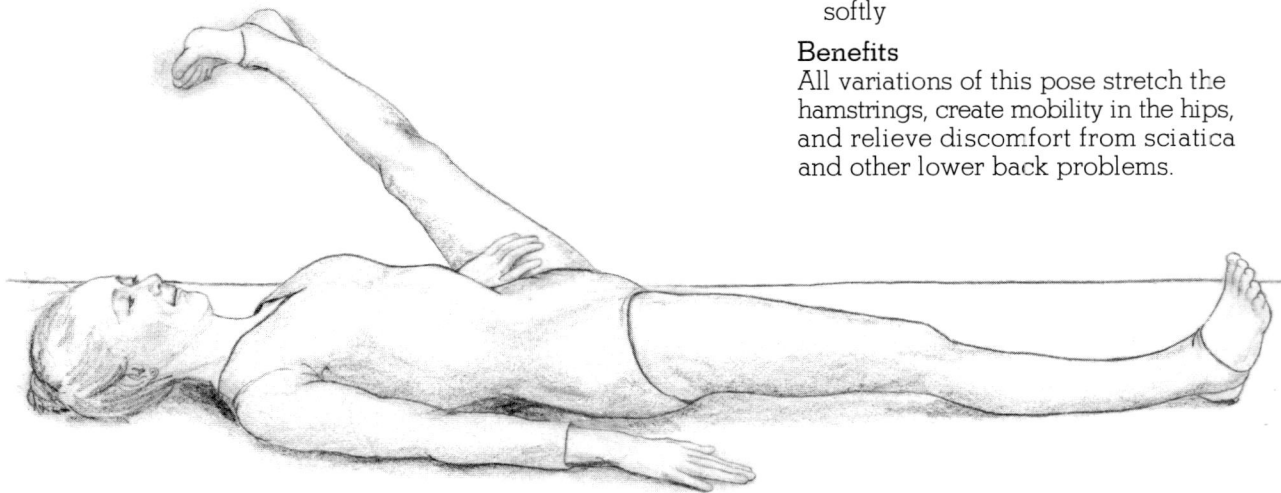

Relaxation: The Corpse Pose

"Shavasana is a great posture. Only the yogis know the mystery of it. After doing other asanas you must lie down in Shavasana, *otherwise your practice of yoga will not bear fruit. At one time, I practiced all the asanas, and afterwards I would always lie in* Shavasana *to get rid of the fatigue which came from the other asanas. After meditation one should do* Shavasana *for a few minutes also. In that way the elements and cells of the body that become disturbed during meditation return to normal. If you find sitting in a cross-legged posture for meditation very difficult, you can lie in* Shavasana *and meditate. You can practice this even when going to sleep at night. If you repeat the mantra, after some time you will find that the mantra will continue on its own throughout the night, and you will be aware of it when you wake up in the morning."*

—Swami Muktananda

SHAVASANA
(*shava*, corpse; corpse pose)

This posture is recommended for complete mental and physical relaxation. It should be practiced for 5 to 10 minutes at the end of each asana session, and both before and after any breathing exercises.

Lie on your back, and check the position of the head. If it tilts back, place a cushion or folded blanket under the head, so that forehead and chin are on the same level.

- extend legs fully and lengthen lower back toward heels
- separate legs a few inches, and allow feet to fall naturally to sides
- turn upper arms out, slightly away from the torso, with palms facing up
- relax each portion of body separately, beginning with feet and moving gradually upwards to head and face
- focus on the breath, or repeat the mantra (as described in the section on Siddha Meditation)

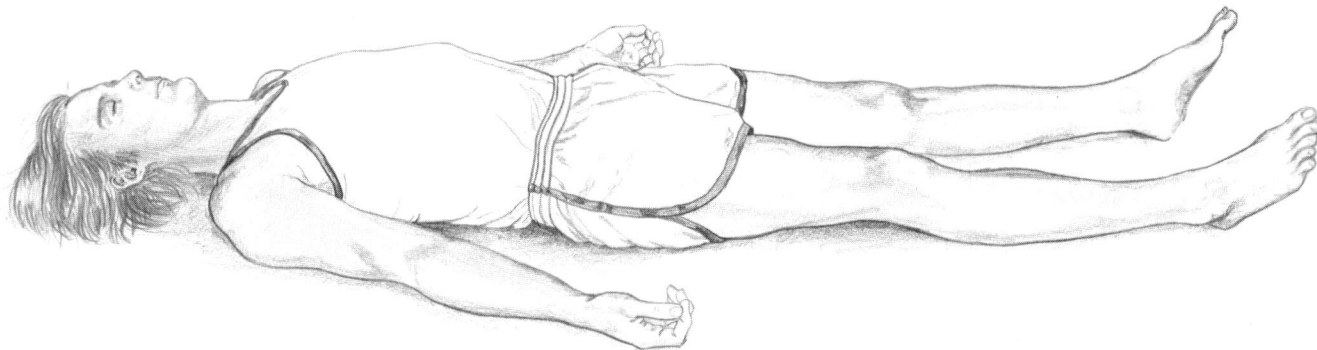

FULL YOGIC BREATH

This technique corrects shallow breathing by encouraging maximum movement of the lungs, thereby expanding their capacity for inhaling and exhaling. Generally, our breathing is restricted to the upper chest area. This is the result of inner tension, which causes the abdominal muscles to tighten.

Full yogic breathing brings an increased supply of oxygen to the lungs, blood, heart and brain. This has an extremely beneficial effect on the nervous system and can be immediately experienced as an increased sense of peace and well-being. Prana, the vital life force that moves throughout the body and intermingles with the breath, is very closely linked to the mind, which is why the yogis use the practice of pranayama, breath control, as a prelude to meditation. Through pranayama the prana is purified and the mind and nerves are refined, which enables a meditator to experience higher states of meditation.

The Full Yogic Breath helps to develop control of the abdominal muscles, and increases breathing capacity, both essential for *Bhastrika*, the breathing technique Swami Muktananda recommended as an aid to the practice of meditation.

The best time to practice the Full Yogic Breath is first thing in the morning, when the lungs are fresh and the body fully rested. Be sure to lie in *Shavasana* for a few minutes before you do any breathing excercises; when you are finished with the exercises, lie in *Shavasana* again, in order to allow the breathing rhythm to return to normal. If you want to practice the Full Yogic Breath immediately after the postures, you should relax in *Shavasana* for 5-10 minutes before beginning the deep breathing. By combining relaxation and full breathing with the performance of the asanas, you will eliminate fatigue and feel re-energized.

FULL YOGIC BREATH

Preparation: The Full Yogic Breath is composed of three phases. Practice the three phases separately until you can successfully combine them into one complete breath. Remember to breathe through the nostrils with the mouth closed.

Lie on your back.

PART 1/ABDOMINAL BREATHING

- first, exhale completely
- relax abdominal muscles, focus attention on abdomen
- inhaling, expand abdominal muscles
- exhaling, relax and gently contract abdominal muscles

Continue this first phase until it becomes smooth and effortless. Check the movement by placing your hand below the navel.

PART 2/MIDDLE CHEST BREATHING

- first, exhale completely
- inhaling, expand rib cage
- exhaling, release rib cage

To check movement, place backs of fingers against sides of rib cage, and apply gentle pressure.

PART 3/UPPER CHEST BREATHING

- first, exhale completely
- inhaling, widen collarbones
- exhaling, release upper chest

To check this movement, place your hand on the upper chest, just below the collarbones.

FULL YOGIC BREATH

Instructions

Lie on your back.

- first, exhale completely
- slowly inhaling, expand abdomen, then rib cage, then widen upper chest
- slowly exhaling, release abdomen, then rib cage, and then the upper chest

As soon as you expand the rib cage, the abdomen will become slightly contracted. A flowing, steady movement is essential to the successful performance of this breathing technique; this will be achieved with practice.

BHASTRIKA

This is called *Shambhavi Bhastrika* because Lord Shiva first taught this technique to the Goddess Shambhavi. It has tremendous value and is highly mysterious. It destroys all diseases, particularly the diseases of the stomach. When you do *Bhastrika*, your stomach ailments will vanish, and your appetite will increase a lot. Not only that, the essence of food will permeate your entire system more effectively. Your stomach will become very flat, and all bad gases will be expelled. You will be filled with fresh oxygen, and the prana will be purified. Your brain will become strengthened, and your Kundalini will awaken very quickly if you practice *Bhastrika* in a proper manner.

The effect of *Bhastrika* is very intense, so you must be strong and absolutely disciplined to practice it. You can't break the discipline of this technique, even in the smallest way. If something has great power, it can also be harmful. Fire is great; it helps to cook food and give warmth. Nonetheless, if you break the discipline and stick your hands in the fire, you'll get burned. So one who wishes to derive benefit from the practice of *Bhastrika* must observe certain discipline.

First of all, you should learn it from a very good teacher, one who has learned it perfectly. Then to do *Bhastrika* you should sit in a good posture, either *Padmasana, Siddha-sana*, or *Sukhasana*. Your spine must be straight. The head, the heart and the base of the spine should be in a straight line. Beginners can sit against a wall to keep their backs straight. Place your hands in *Chin Mudra* (with thumb and index finger touching) on your knees. Your mind should be quiet, and you must have an empty stomach. You should wait at least two hours after eating before doing *Bhastrika*, and wait another hour after doing it before eating again. You should do this technique in the open air, if possible, where the air is fresh, but if it is too cold, you can do it in your room before you sit for meditation. In the beginning you might find it difficult to do, but continue to practice with discipline and after a while it will come to you very easily. Increase the duration of *Bhastrika* very slowly. Afterwards, lie down in *Shavasana* quietly for five minutes until the prana becomes quiet and still, and then you can sit for meditation.

Swami Muktananda

BHASTRIKA

Bhastrika pranayama is a breathing technique in which the abdominal muscles are forcibly expanded and contracted to regulate inhalation and exhalation. The abdomen expands with the inbreath and contracts with the outbreath. The breathing is a short, rapid movement in and out through the nose. The action is to draw the breath in quickly through the nostrils with some force, then immediately expel it, in a manner similar to a strong, quick blowing of the nose. The emphasis on inhaling and exhaling is equal. Once you master the practice of *Bhastrika*, the breath will be regulated by abdominal muscle movement only; the rest of the body will remain still. If you practice it incorrectly, by contracting the higher muscles of the stomach rather than those of the lower abdomen, you may experience nausea or unpleasant dizziness, accompanied by a cold sweat. Focus on using only the abdominal muscles; the stomach may move a little, sympathetically, but it is not involved in activating the breathing. Your ability to control the correct muscles will improve with regular practice of the Full Yogic Breath.

Swami Muktananda strongly recommended that one not begin the practice of *Bhastrika* without the guidance of a reliable teacher. The following directions are not meant to replace formal instruction, but to serve as a reminder of the correct technique. It is essential that you check your technique with your teacher before regularly practicing *Bhastrika*.

BHASTRIKA
(*bhastrika*: bellows; bellows breathing)

Sit in *Padmasana, Ardha Padmasana, Swastikasana* or *Sukhasana*. If you cannot sit in one of these postures, use *Vajrasana*, with knees widespread.

- place hands on knees in *Chin Mudra* (thumb and index finger touching)
- lift pelvis and spine, and relax shoulders
- keep head and neck straight
- focus attention on breath
- begin rapid breathing with a forceful exhalation
- continue for as long as possible up to a maximum of 40 breaths
- on final exhalation, contract abdomen forcefully, expelling all air
- inhale, using Full Yogic Breath
- retain breath for as long as is comfortable
- exhale, using Full Yogic Breath
- this constitutes one round

Begin with 5 rounds. After practicing regularly for one month, increase to 10 rounds. Increase beyond 10 rounds only with permission from your teacher.

Caution
Bhastrika should not be done by pregnant women, or by people with heart problems or high blood pressure. Discontinue practicing *Bhastrika* if you experience pressure in the eyes, pain in the ears, or nose bleeds.

Mastery of an asana is essential for everyone who wishes to meditate. It is the foundation of yoga. You cannot get into an advanced state of meditation if your posture is not firm and steady. Not only that, you cannnot even enjoy good health. I am using the word "health" in a yogic sense. The yogic concept of health is quite different from the ordinary concept of health. If you can sit in one position without moving for three hours, all of the *nadis*, subtle nerves in the body, are purified, the blocks in the nerves are removed, the *prana* is strengthened, and the body creates medicine for different diseases within. The mind also becomes very strong, the intellect becomes very sharp, and happiness also increases. The *Shiva Sutras* of Kashmir Shaivism say, "One who has mastered a meditative posture enjoys the inner happiness welling up spontaneously in his heart." Therefore, posture is of the greatest importance in the practice of yoga. Once your sitting posture becomes firm, your mind will become steady. Your mind is restless and wandering only so long as your posture is not firm.

In the beginning it may be difficult for you to sit cross-legged. However, don't be in a hurry; do it gradually. On the first day practice sitting in a meditative posture for one minute, sitting totally still. The second day sit for two minutes like that, and the third day for three minutes. Within a month you will be able to sit still for half an hour.

After two months you will be able to sit still for one hour. When you can sit completely still for one hour, without moving, understand that you have become fifty percent a yogi. The true sign of a yogi is not that he gives high philosophical lectures. A true yogi should be able to sit completely still for one, two, three hours. The longer you can sit still on the outside without moving at all, the stiller the mind becomes. It is not at all necessary for one who can sit absolutely still in a posture for two or three hours to practice *pranayama* or *samadhi*, because both will come to him by themselves.

The yoga scriptures such as *Gheranda Samhita* and Patanjali's *Yoga Sutras* mention 84 asanas. Among those classical asanas, three are the most important for meditation: *Padmasana, Siddhasana* and *Sukhasana.*

Padmasana is a great posture. It has enormous value. When you sit in the lotus posture the 720,000,000 *nadis* are purified. Diseases are caused by impurities in the *nadis*, and when these *nadis* are purified, the body functions very well.

If you cannot sit in *Padmasana*, you can sit in *Sukhasana* — a posture that is easy and comfortable.

Whichever posture you sit in, you must keep your back straight. The base of the spine, the back of the neck, and the top of the head should be completely straight.

It is also good to keep your hands on the knees in the *Chin Mudra*, with the thumb and the first finger held together. The secret of this *mudra* is that it stops the outward flow of the inner energy, and it also helps you to achieve one-pointedness of mind in meditation.

—*Swami Muktananda*

Meditation Postures

1. Choose a meditation posture which allows you to sit comfortably with the spine erect.

2. For cross-legged poses, place a cushion or folded blanket under the sitting bones, so that the pelvis is lifted vertically, and both knees are in contact with the floor, if possible.

3. Never try to force your legs into a position, as an injury can result very easily to the ligaments and the tendons of the knee. Such injuries take many months to heal.

4. If you experience knee pain, try placing a small rolled cloth behind the knee to create space in the joint. If this does not alleviate the pain, choose an easier posture.

5. Rememeber to change the cross of your legs at regular intervals. If you sit for long periods of time with the legs always crossed in the same direction, one hip becomes much tighter than the other, and the spinal column is imbalanced.

6. Adjust your weight evenly between the right hip and the left hip. Bring the center of the shoulders directly over the center of the hips. Feel that the whole spinal column is balanced lightly on the firm foundation of the pelvis. With this inner balance and inner lightness, meditation progresses rapidly.

SUKHASANA
(*sukha*: ease; easy posture)

According to the *Yoga Sutras*, any posture that can be held steadily and comfortably may be called *Sukhasana*. However, it generally refers to this simple cross-legged posture, which is suitable for meditation.

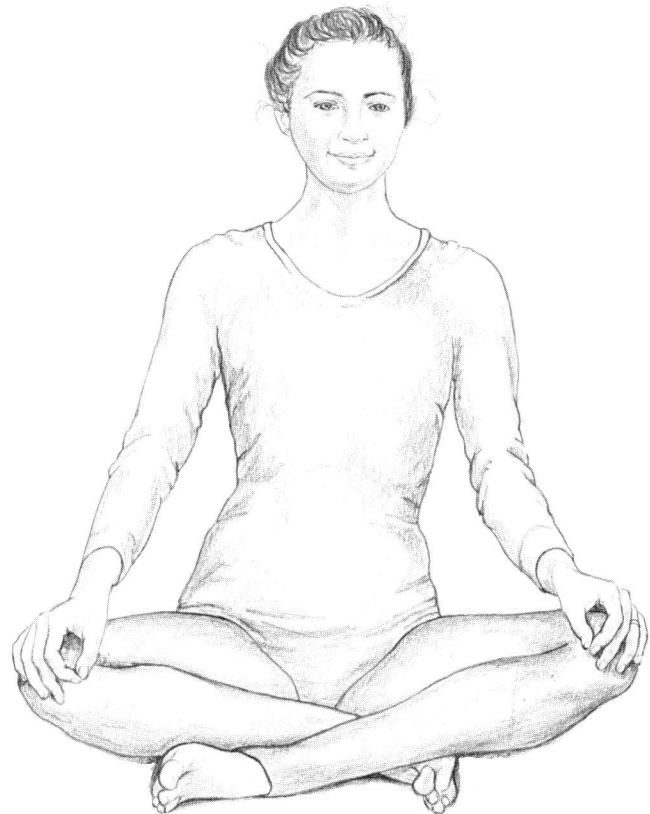

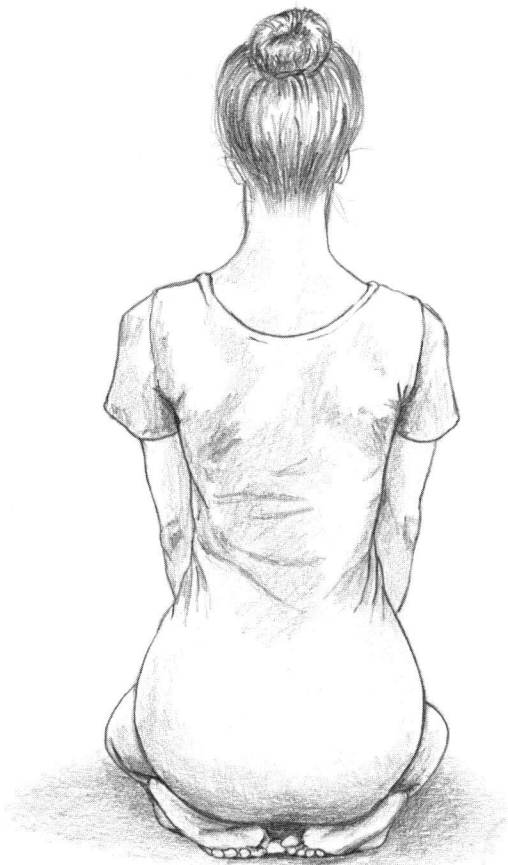

VAJRASANA

(*vajra*: thunderbolt; thunderbolt pose)

Sit on your heels.

- separate heels, bring big toes together
- rest buttocks on insides of feet
- knees remain together
- place hands on knees
- lift pelvis and lengthen spine

For comfort, a small pillow or folded blanket may be placed on the heels. If necessary, a thick cushion or blanket can be placed between the feet in order to elevate the body and avoid strain to ankles and knees.

Benefits

If *Vajrasana* is held for fifteen minutes after eating, it aids digestion. It also helps to steady the mind. People with sciatica should substitute this posture for cross-legged positions.

SWASTIKASANA
(*swastika*: auspicious; auspicious pose)

Sit cross-legged on a blanket or cushion.

- place feet beneath thighs, with soles touching thighs
- tuck toes of each foot between calf and thigh muscles
- knees should touch floor

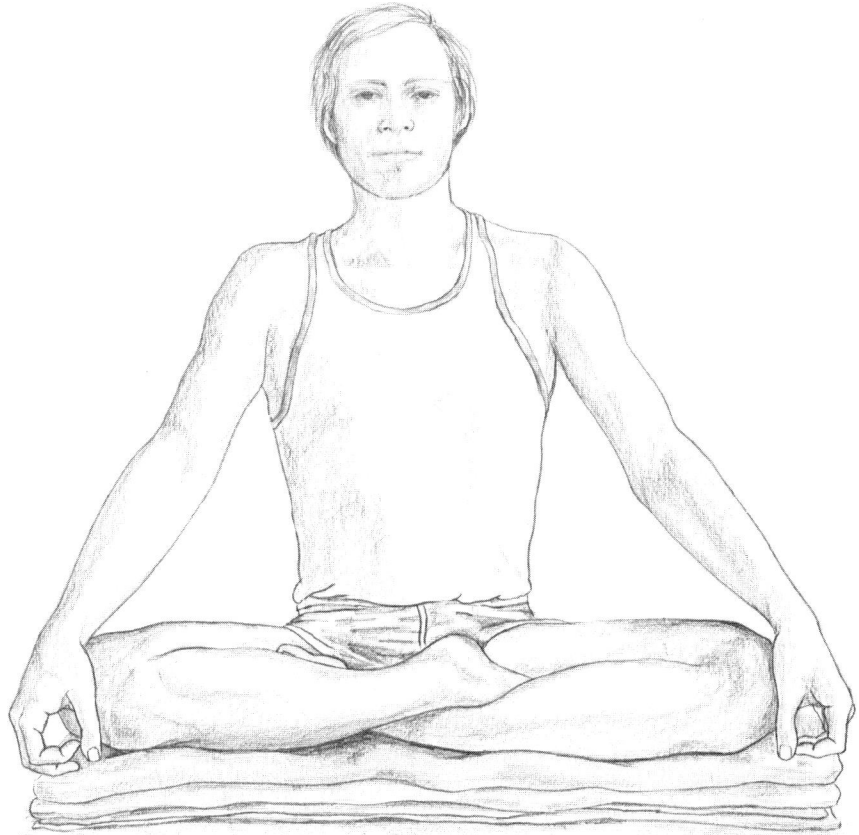

ARDHA PADMASANA

(*ardha*: half, *padma*, lotus; half-lotus posture)

Before attempting to sit in *Ardha Padmasana* for any length of time, you should master *Baddha Konasana*, that is, sitting with the soles of the feet together, and the thighs and knees in contact with the floor.

Sit at the edge of a blanket or cushion with the legs outstretched.

- place left foot beneath right thigh
- draw right foot to top of left thigh
- both knees should contact floor — if not, you need a higher blanket under hips

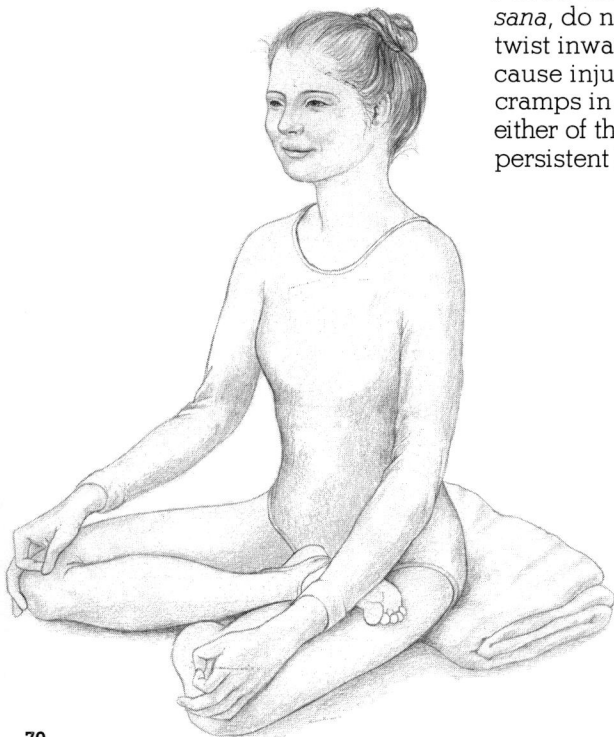

PADMASANA

(*padma*: lotus; lotus posture)

Before attempting to sit in *Padmasana*, you should master *Ardha Padmasana* and *Baddha Konasana* (sitting with the soles of the feet together, and the thighs and knees in contact with the floor).

Sit with the legs outstretched.

- place right foot on root of left thigh
- bend left knee, lift leg by holding under shin, and place left foot on right thigh

Caution

For *Ardha Padmasana* and *Padmasana*, do not allow the feet to sickle or twist inwards at the ankle, as this may cause injury to the outer knee and cramps in the feet. Do not remain in either of these poses if you experience persistent knee pain.

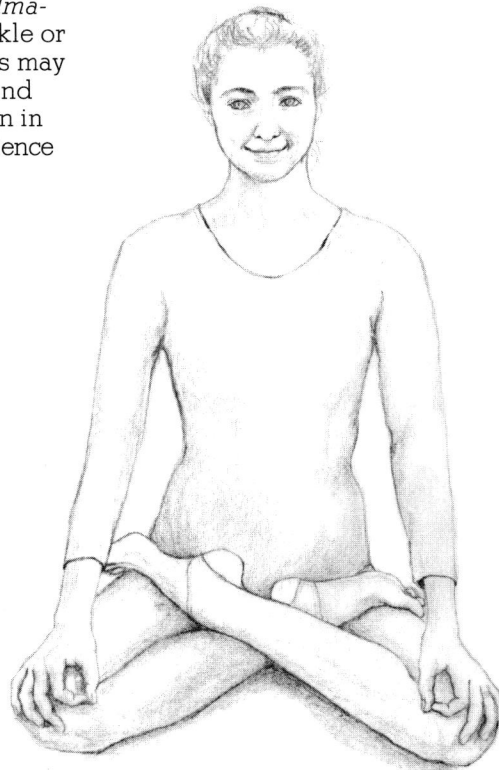

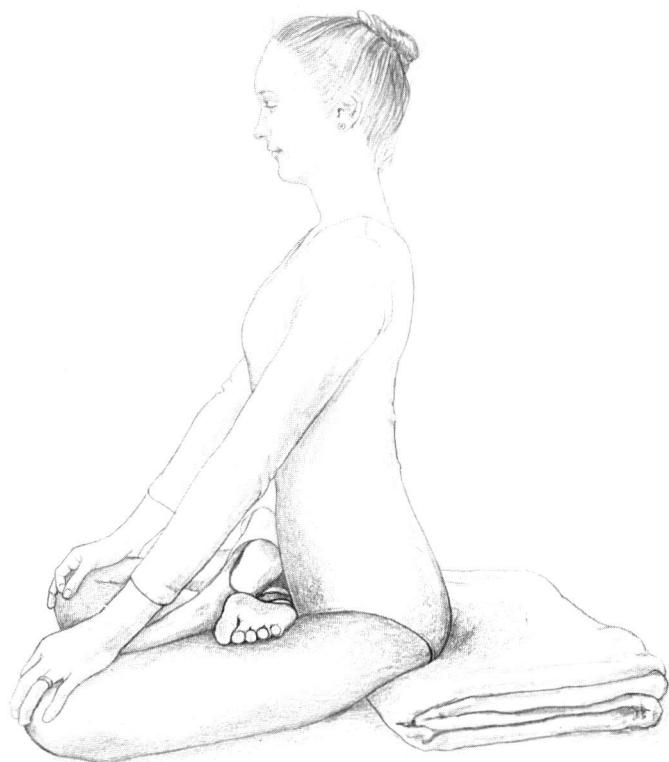

A great sage, Patanjali, wrote a treatise called the *Yoga Sutras*. In the first aphorism, he describes yoga as: *Yogash chitta vritti nirodhah*—"Yoga is to still the tendencies of the mind." Yoga consists not just of performing asanas or pranayama, but of making the mind quiet. When the mind becomes still then one enters into meditation. Patanjali goes on to say: "Meditation is to become free from mentation." There should be no thoughts in the mind; it should be completely empty. That is meditation, and when that occurs, the inner yoga begins to take place.

When one starts to meditate with success, one's inner Shakti is awakened and the process of inner purification begins. As the mind becomes purified through meditation, bliss arises from within, and the movement of prana becomes regulated. In our present condition, when the mind is agitated and distracted the movement of prana is not smooth; it is jerky and disturbed. As a result, we suffer from different ailments and a lack of peace. Meditation promotes longevity, because it brings the body into a state of perfect balance, perfect equipoise. All the body's deficiencies and excesses are corrected, and oxygen is distributed evenly to all its parts. In meditation, the needs of the entire body are attended to by the awakened Kundalini energy.

Meditation transforms you into a veritable abode of love, peace, and bliss. Through proper meditation, you will overcome all negative tendencies— passions, jealousy, hatred and hostility toward others. Meditation will make you aware of the divine inner power, Kundalini Shakti. Due to ignorance of this power, we consider ourselves to be small, insecure and limited. Through meditation we become aware of our inherent greatness.

Meditation is such a great purifier that it washes away the sins of countless lifetimes and removes all the impurities and tensions which beset the mind. Meditation rids us of disease and makes us more skillful in everything we do. Through meditation, our inner awareness expands and our understanding of inner and outer things becomes steadily deeper. Through meditation, we travel to different inner worlds and have innumerable inner experiences. Above all, meditation stills the mind, which constantly wanders and causes suffering, and establishes us forever in the state of supreme peace which is independent of any external factors. Ultimately, meditation makes us aware of our own true nature. It is this awareness which removes all suffering and delusion, and this awareness manifests only when we come face to face with our own inner Self.

Four factors are involved in Siddha meditation: the object of meditation, which is the inner Self; the mantra, which is the vibration of the Self; the asana, or posture, in which we can sit comfortably for a long time; and the natural pranayama, which arises when we repeat the mantra with love and reverence. These four factors are interrelated and when they come together, meditation occurs in a very natural manner.

The first question which arises when you sit for meditation is, "On what should I meditate?" Yogis meditate on many kinds of objects and recommend many different techniques. Maharshi Patanjali speaks of concentration, or *dharana*, in which one focuses one's attention on a particular object in order to still and focus the mind. You can concentrate on the heart or on the space between the eyebrows; or you can focus your mind on a great being who has risen above attachment and aversion, who has destroyed the sense of duality. The mind becomes whatever it contemplates, whatever it takes interest in and loves.

Many people complain to me, "Baba, whenever I sit for meditation my mind begins to wander. It wanders here, it wanders there, and it doesn't listen to me." I ask, "Why are you meditating on the mind?" Meditate on the one who is the knower of the mind. Think of the one who is totally free and who knows everything, and everyone, from within. Meditate on the one who is aware of the wandering, the unsteadiness and the restlessness of your mind. Meditate on that. Do not meditate on the wanderings of the mind. The inner knower is in meditation even when the mind is wandering; that Self is constantly observing the mind. Your goal is not to battle with the mind, but to witness the mind. Know that you are the witness, the Self, and let the mind go wherever it likes.

If you still cannot meditate, then you can take the help of a mantra. Mantra is the very life of meditation, the greatest of all techniques. Mantra is a cosmic word or sound vibration. It is the vibration of the Self, the true speech of the Self, and when we immerse ourselves in it, it leads us to the place of the Self. As we repeat the mantra, we should focus our attention within, on the place which is the source of the mantra. As we repeat the mantra more and more, it penetrates the entire territory of our mind and purifies it completely. The secret of mantra repetition is that, when you repeat it, you are repeating your own name. If

you repeat it with the understanding that the mantra is the vibration of the Self, it will give you the experience of that innermost Consciousness.

Another important factor in meditation is the sitting posture, or asana. The asana is the foundation on which the entire structure of yoga rests. The *Yoga Sutras* say that the correct sitting posture is that in which one can sit comfortably for a long time. You can use either *Siddhasana*, *Padmasana*, or *Sukhasana* for meditation. Or, if you cannot sit comfortably in any of these, you can lie down in *Shavasana* and meditate in that position. Sitting in a proper posture, however, with the spine straight, enables the mind to turn inward, and then meditation will come easily.

The final factor in meditation is pranayama, the breathing process. Some yogis practice different kinds of pranayama, and they do it so much that they ruin their minds, their intellects, and their bodies. If you want to practice a few asanas and *Bhastrika* before you meditate, it will be beneficial, provided that you have learned the technique correctly from a qualified teacher. But when you sit for meditation, the breathing process should be natural and spontaneous; you should not try to disturb the natural rhythm of the breath.

Once the Kundalini is awakened, different types of breathing techniques may occur spontaneously during meditation. Sometimes the breath becomes slow or sometimes very rapid and forceful, or the breath may become suspended; this depends upon the working of the Shakti within. Do not try to control the breath, but let these changes occur spontaneously. In the meantime, if you can, combine the mantra with your breath: repeat it once with the inbreath and once with the outbreath. The mind and prana are connected, so that when the prana becomes steady, the mind also becomes steady. Therefore, if the mind becomes focused on the mantra or the breath, it becomes calm. Then the prana is automatically stabilized.

If you combine these different means with faith in the Guru's teachings, your inner Shakti will unfold. Then all kinds of kriyas, or yogic movements, will take place. Do not be frightened by them; they are all a play of the inner Shakti, and they will work to purify the body and the mind. Diseases will be cured, and addictions will fall away by themselves. As the mind is purified, your entire life will be purified. This is how the awakened Shakti works. Once it is activated, your spiritual journey begins. The Shakti ensures good meditation, which brings about experiences on all levels, ultimately giving you the knowledge of your true being. The veil of ignorance obscuring your true nature is removed, and you are able to see yourself and the world in true perspective. You attain divine vision, so that you no longer see this world as filled with duality and diversity. Instead of seeing differences between man and woman, or East and West, you will understand that the entire universe is an expansion of your own Self. You will realize that everything is a play of Consciousness and that, just as the bubbles and waves of the ocean arise and subside in the ocean, whatever exists arises and subsides in the Self.

Just as you slip easily into sleep, you should be able to slip easily into meditation. Sit peacefully, be with yourself. Focus your mind on the inner Consciousness, the inner knower. Let your breath move naturally and watch it — do not force anything. Become immersed in your own inner Self. Turn your mind and senses inward. If thoughts arise, let them come and go. Watch the source of your thoughts. Meditate with the awareness that you are the witness of the mind. True meditation is to become free from mentation. The moment the thoughts become still, the light of the Self will shine from within. However, if the mind does not immediately become thoughtfree, do not try to erase the thoughts forcibly. Respect the mind and understand that, whatever comes and goes within, it is a form of the Self. Then it will automatically become still.

To help quiet the mind, you may take the support of the mantra; repeat either *Om Namah Shivaya* or *So'ham*. Both mantras are one; both come from the Self. Only the method of repeating them differs. *Om Namah Shivaya* means, "I bow to the Lord, who is the inner Self." Repeat it silently, along with your breath, or at the same rate of speed at which you speak. Repeat it with love, and go deep inside.

If you wish to practice the *So'ham* mantra with complete understanding of the significance of this natural mantra, you should read *I Am That*. *So'ham* means "I am That (Supreme Consciousness)," and it repeats itself spontaneously with every breath. Become aware of the sound of your breath. As you inhale, the sound is *ham*; as you exhale, the sound is *so*. Perceive the space where *ham* merges inside, before *so* arises. Perceive the space where *so* merges outside, before *ham* arises. This space of stillness, the space between the breaths, is the space of the Self. Focus on that space and you will naturally experience the Self.

Lose yourself in meditation. No matter what feeling arises, let it be. The inner energy is filled with infinite techniques, processes, and feelings, and its play is in everything. Therefore, everything belongs to it, and it is one with your Self.

The purpose of meditation is inner happiness, inner peace. When all the senses become quiet and you experience bliss, that is the attainment. The world is the embodiment of joy; joy lives everywhere. Find it, and attain it. Instead of having negative thoughts, have the awareness "I am pure; I am joy." Feel good about yourself — fill yourself with great divinity.

Become quiet with the awareness that everything is you and you are everything.

Meditate on your Self. Honor your Self. Understand your Self. God dwells within you, as you.

—Swami Muktananda

Q: What is Siddha Yoga, and how is it different from other yogas?
SM: Siddha Yoga is a technique which expands the spiritual energy. Within every person there is a hidden divine force, and the means of awakening that force is called *shaktipat.* In Siddha Yoga, *shaktipat,* or initiation, takes place through four means: through the touch, look word or thought of a Siddha Guru. Once your inner power is awakened by grace, it automatically takes you to higher and higher levels of experience, until you reach a state of equanimity. In other yogas, you have to exert yourself a lot; you have to do so many practices, and even then a seeker rarely becomes centered in the superconscious or highest state. However, Siddha Yoga brings perfection to you. Also, it is a spontaneous yoga. It takes place even while you go about your work in the world. After you receive this grace from the Guru, and the inner Shakti is awakened, everything happens spontaneously.

Q: Do you need a Guru to awaken the inner energy?
SM: To awaken the Shakti, or inner energy, it is absolutely essential to consult someone who is capable of awakening it within you. No matter what you want to accomplish in life, you first have to learn from someone who has already accomplished it. In the same way, to accomplish the awakening, you must learn from an adept Master. Then, once the Shakti is awakened, the Shakti itself becomes the Master, guiding the student from within. Your own inner Shakti will direct you until you reach the state of perfection. At the end of your journey you will come to know that you are perfect, and that you were always perfect. The Guru is needed to point out to you the perfection that has been with you all along.

Q: Is it necessary for me to be able to do all the asanas before I can make any significant progress?
SM: Asanas are meant for physical purification. If you practice asanas, your progress in meditation will be quicker. Otherwise, for the purification which would have been brought about by asanas, you would have to meditate for a very long time. In meditation, your body will be purified, but you will not be able to advance very fast. Asanas purify the nerves and thus ensure a smooth flow of prana through them. In meditation, the prana should be able to flow freely throughout the body, from head to toe. When its movement becomes smooth, supreme peace arises up from within, and you do not need to make an effort with your mind, again and again, to become balanced. The sages say that when the prana begins to flow quickly throughout the body, one obtains the vision of equality and tranquility. I was very fat at one time, and it was practicing asanas that helped me to slim down.

Q: I have heard you tell people not to do the headstand. Could you explain why?
SM: The headstand is not suitable for everybody. To know whether it is suitable for you, you have to be checked by a very good yogi or Ayurvedic doctor who can tell you which humor is predominant in your system. If you have too much bile in your body, then it is terrible for you. People who have too much bile are very thin; their bodies are warm and their heads are hot. Such people should never do the headstand, because a tremendous amount of heat is created, then it affects the brain. People with predominant wind or phlegm in their bodies can do it, but they should be very disciplined in the practice. Everyone can do *Sarvangasana,* the shoulderstand, and obtain the same benefits.

Q: Should one meditate when he is ill?
SM: It is good to meditate during illness, because meditation will help you get over it quickly. If you meditate calmly, either in the sitting or lying position, meditation will help you overcome the illness or, if there is pain in any part of the body, meditation will drive it away. However, if you are ill, you should not practice asanas or pranayama, particularly *Bhastrika;* but meditation can be practiced in all conditions.

Q: Should I have a special place for meditation?

SM: It is very good to set aside a place for meditation. If it is possible, have a special room but, if not, a corner will do. Purify it by chanting God's name, and try not to let anything take place there which will disturb its atmosphere. In the place where you meditate regularly, the vibrations of meditation gather, and after a while it becomes very easy to meditate there. For the same reason, you should set aside special clothes and a mat for meditation; do not wash them too often, because the Shakti will accumulate in them and make it easy for you to meditate.

If possible, meditate at the same time every day. The early hours of the morning between 3 a.m. and 6 a.m., are best for meditation, but you can meditate at any time which is convenient. If you become accustomed to meditating at a certain hour, your body will develop the habit of meditation. I have been meditating every morning at 3 a.m. for many years and, even now, my body automatically goes into meditation at that hour.

Q: How long should one wait after eating to meditate, practice Hatha Yoga or sleep?

SM: Immediately after eating, you will not be able to meditate very well, because the Shakti is not able to circulate freely when the stomach is full of food. So it is not good to meditate while food is still in the stomach. Meditate before you eat, or at least two hours after eating.

For all yogic practices, the stomach should be completely empty. Those who practice or teach Hatha Yoga should know that one must not practice asanas for at least three hours after a meal; also, one must not eat or drink anything for at least one half hour after a session of Hatha Yoga. A teacher of Hatha Yoga should make sure his students know this.

The sages have said that we should eat food in the same way that we take medicine, regularly and in carefully measured amounts. To ensure proper digestion, you should fill half of your stomach with food, and one quarter with water; the remaining quarter should be left empty, to allow the digestive prana to circulate freely. This way of eating is the sign of a true yogi and is also conducive to living life happily. I read an article about a medical conference at which a famous doctor was asked how much food a person should consume in one day. The doctor replied, "One should eat no more than four hundred grams of food each day. If you eat more than that, you will not be eating for your health, but for your doctor's wealth!" Therefore, exercise control in eating.

You must wait at least two and a half hours before going to sleep, so that the food is at least partially digested. The Jains, a religious sect in India, have a rule that one should not eat after sunset. At first, I thought the rule was absurd, but when I thought carefully about it, I saw that there was some sense in it. What usually happens is that we delay our dinner because of gossiping, and then we eat rather late and go to sleep right after dinner. If you eat before sunset, it ensures that at least three or four hours will pass before you go to bed.

Q: What do you have to say about proper diet? For example, is it wrong to eat meat?

SM: I do not say that you must not eat meat, but you do not need it for meditation. In meditation, the inner energy first purifies your body. By eating meat, you are making the body impure again; so there is more work for the energy to do. If you want to reach higher stages of meditation quickly, it would be better to give up meat. Eat light foods that will give you strength; for example, butter, milk and honey. What meat do those animals eat, whose flesh we eat? They are strictly vegetarian; they live on grass and leaves, so we too can get our strength and flesh through vegetarian foods. I am not against meat eating; however, for meditation, it is necessary that your food be pure. If you were to eat pure food for a while, you would get into higher stages of meditation more quickly.

Q: Why should we limit our meditation to an hour and a half every day?

SM: It is not that you have to limit meditation to only an hour and a half, but you should increase the duration very gradually. Also, the length of time one can meditate is influenced by the strength of one's constitution. If one meditates more than the body can stand, one's head will become too hot. Serious meditators must be sure to eat the right kinds of food. Here in our kitchen, we use cashew and pistachio nuts, clarified butter, raisins, and other such good foods which will give you a lot of strength. There are many different fluids in the body, but the most important one is called *ojas*, a beautiful, shining yellow fluid that is situated in the bone marrow. The *ojas* is created through semen; it is very radiant, and it gives you the power of memory as well as strength. If we meditate too much and do not give enough rich food to our bodies, the fire of meditation begins to consume the *ojas* from our bones, and we become dull, lose enthusiasm, and become very tired. This is why we have a time limit for meditation.

You can meditate six hours a day if you like, but you have to eat good rich food so that you will have sufficient strength. You will also have to remain celibate, because this *ojas* is created by semen.

If you wish, you can meditate twice a day—one hour in the morning and one hour in the evening—provided that you drink milk and eat sweet things, such as fruit or honey. Even though meditation appears to be very ordinary, it has a lot of power in it: it is like a big fire. In the West, people think that meditation is very mundane and simple, but when you meditate, the fire of meditation burns up all the impurities inside you and makes you completely pure. The more you meditate, the more your body is purified, and if you meditate a lot, you can completely rejuvenate your body, no matter how old you may be. Many ancient sages rejuvenated their bodies in this way but, practically speaking, to attain salvation or to experience peace, you do not have to do this. However, your mind should become still, and you should become established in your own inner Self. Meditation purifies all your nerves, all your vital airs and, in due course, it gives a lot of strength to your body. In the beginning, though, it consumes strength.

Q: Some spiritual teachers recommend sex as an aid in the process of spiritual evolution, whereas others say that one should abstain. What is your opinion?

SM: The sexual fluid is very valuable. The stronger the sexual fluid is, and the more it is retained in the body, the purer and more tranquil the mind will be. The more tranquil the mind becomes, the easier it will be for it to turn inward, and it will also acquire the power to make discoveries in the inner realms.

Seekers can be divided into two categories: total celibates and householders. I am not against married life—in ancient times there were many yogis who were married—nor am I against producing children. But one who is interested in making spiritual progress must conserve his sexual fluid.

Q: Herbal remedies are said to be healing for body, mind and spirit. Do you think it is necessary to take these as well as meditating with a mantra?

SM: I have studied Ayurveda, the Indian system of medicine. It deals with herbal remedies. According to Ayurveda, every single plant in the world is a remedy if you know how to use it. We use plants in one form or another every day to keep us healthy, and when we get sick it is because we are not using them properly. All our food is medicine. Onion is a great medicine, so are garlic and coriander. It is good to study the properties of the foods we eat and then eat them properly. We should know when it is good to eat something and when it is not. For instance, when it is cold, it is good to drink hot milk but not to eat yoghurt. So, we should know the properties of what we eat.

There was a great doctor of Ayurveda called Charaka. He has described the properties of all the herbs. He knew so much that even though he lived in India he wrote about the climates of other countries too. His work is enormous and very significant. He had many students who all met one day in a conference. Charaka took the form of a bird and sat in a tree under which the conference was being held. The physicians were discussing the relationship between herbs and diseases and describing complicated methods of transforming the body. Then the bird began to call, "*Korarook,*

korarook, korarook? Who is free from disease, who is free from disease, who is free from disease?"

One physician said that if you had a little brandy in the morning, plenty of fish at lunchtime and a lot of whiskey in the evening, you would never get sick. Another said that you should mix yoghurt with milk and add butter, then drink that and you would never be sick. Another said that you should eat something at least eight times a day, once an hour, and you would never be sick. Another said that if you used drugs you would never be sick; your mind might be ruined but your body would be fine. Another said that you should have as much sex as you could; it would not matter if you lost your radiance and vigor. If you indulged your senses all the time you would never be sick. Another said that you should not have anything to do with meditation; then you would never be sick. You should forget about discipline and self-control, and you would be free from sickness.

Charaka could not believe his ears. He had taught them all for such a long time and this was all they had learned from him. He flew away in despair, and arrived at the bank of a beautiful river where an old house was standing. A rishi lived in that house and he was just returning from a bath in the river. The master, who was still in the form of a bird, called to him, "*Korarook, korarook, korarook*?" The rishi looked up. His name was Vagabhatta and he

was a great disciple of Charaka's; he also wrote a large work. As soon as he heard "*Korarook?*" he had the answer to it: "*Hitabhuk, mitabhuk, ritabhuk.*" These three words contain the three basic principles of health. *Hitabhuk* means that you should not eat anything which is not good for you, which makes you sick, which you cannot digest. *Mitabhuk* means that you must not fill your stomach completely. You should fill it half with food, a quarter with water, and leave it a quarter empty; then the digestive fires will blaze all the time. *Ritabhuk* means that you should eat things which suit the season. If it is a cold night and you eat a lot of ice cream, followed by yoghurt, and you wake up the next morning with the flu, it would not be surprising, because this is incompatible with the season.

A person who follows these three principles will always be healthy.

Eat frugally, leave part of your stomach empty at every meal, chew your food well and meditate, and then you will stay perfectly healthy. Food should be light and easily digested. When you get up after a meal you should not feel that you have got a heavy load in your stomach. This is how you should eat. Follow these principles and you will live a healthy, happy and long life.

Q: How will we know if, and when, our Kundalini is awakened?

SM: You will know it. Right now you know that your Kundalini is not awakened. So, if it is awakened you will know it. It has many different effects. Sometimes you become extremely happy, or you feel pressure in the head; you can feel intoxicated, or you can get upset. You can become either very depressed or restless. Do not become scared if these things happen; all are due to the awakening of the Kundalini.

SUGGESTED ROUTINE FOR POSTURES

When you begin practicing Hatha Yoga, start with 15 to 20 minutes per day, and increase the time very gradually. Even if you practice for only a few minutes each day on a regular basis the benefits will be substantial.

The following suggested routines are a guideline to help you plan your daily practices. Alternate programs and include other postures according to your specific needs.

1. Surya Namaskar
   Vidalasana
   Tadasana
   Vrikshasana
   Trikonasana
   Prasarita Padottanasana
   Virasana
   Baddha Konasana
   Janushirshasana
   Paschimottanasana
   Shavasana
   Full Yogic Breath

2. Surya Namaskar
   Konasana
   Parsvakonasana
   Virabhadrasana II
   Uttanasana
   Gomukhasana
   Bharadvajasana
   Baddha Konasana
   Janushirshasana
   Upavistha Konasana
   Jatara Parivartanasana
   Shavasana

3. Surya Namaskar
   Dynamic Plow Movement
   Trikonasana
   Parsvottanasana
   Ardha Chandrasana
   Padangusthasana
   Setu Bandhasana
   Sarvangasana
   Halasana
   Pavana Muktasana
   Supta Padangusthasana
   Shavasana

4. Surya Namaskar
   Konasana
   Parsvakonasana
   Virabhadrasana I
   Uttana Padasana
   Shalabhasana
   Dhanurasana
   Ardha Matsyendrasana
   Marichyasana
   Mandukasana
   Shavasana
   Full Yogic Breath

Appendix B

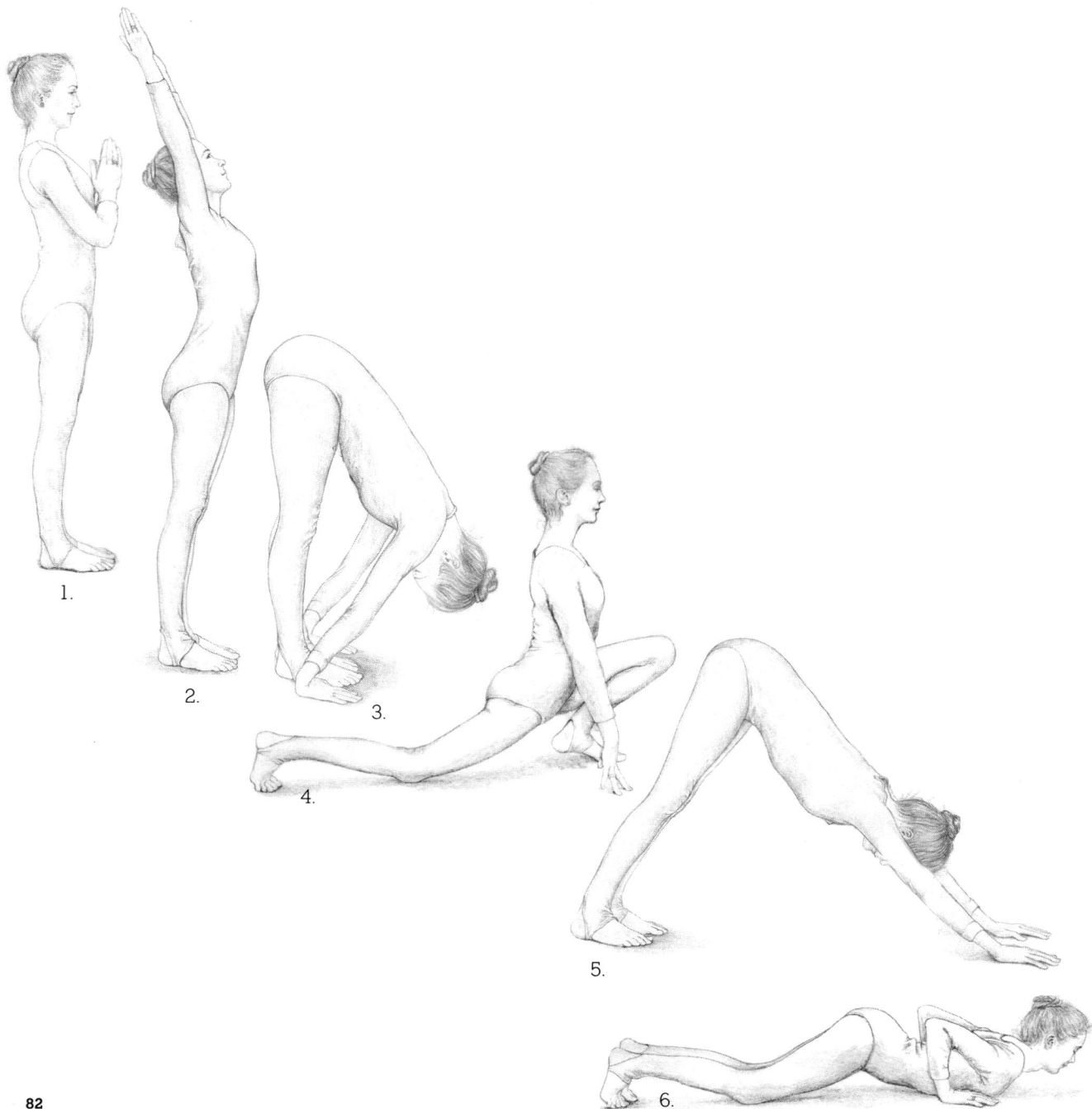

1.

2.

3.

4.

5.

6.

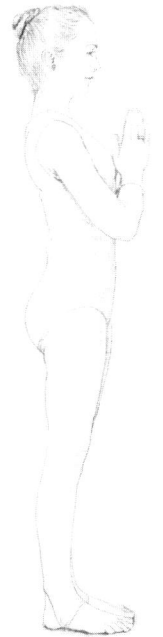

12.

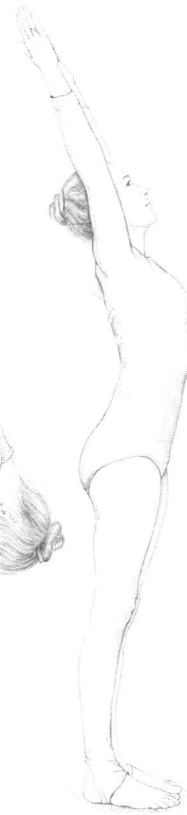

11.

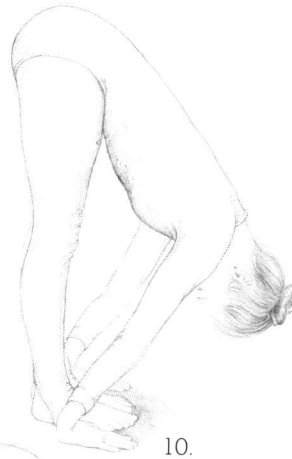

10.

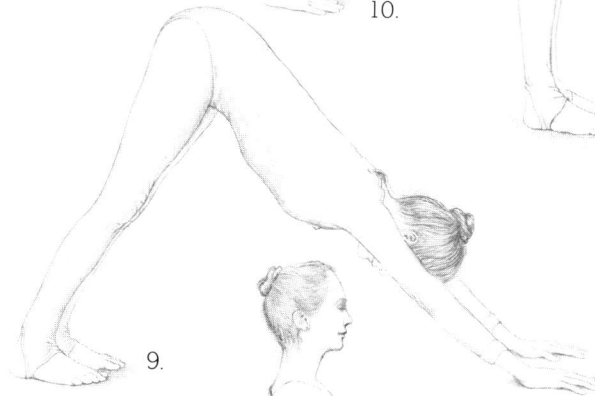

9.

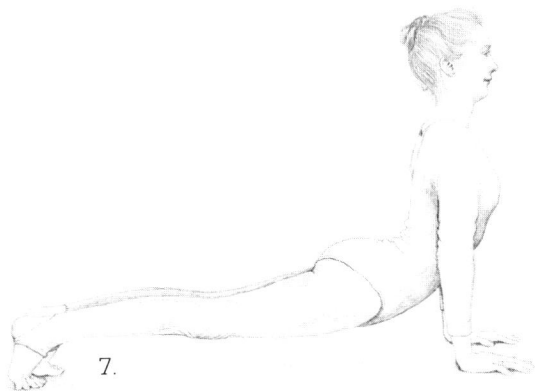

7.

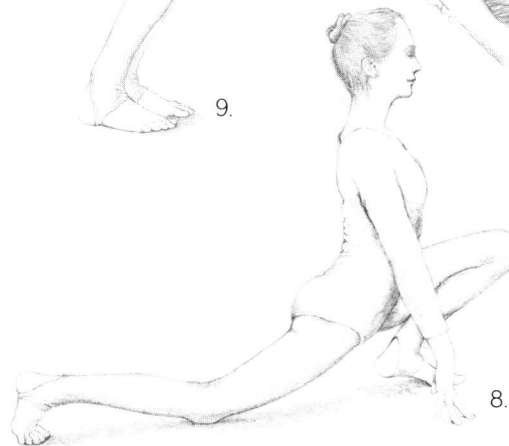

8.

Index

Abdomen, 36, 54; after childbirth, 54; muscles of, 40, 54, 55, 61, 64; organs of, 22, 23, 24, 27, 33, 36, 37, 40, 42, 44, 46, 51, 52, 53, 54, 56; relieving pain in, 23. *See also* Digestion; Intestines
Addictions, 73
Adho Mukha Svanasana, 7, 14
Ankles, 30
Appetite, 37, 63
Ardha Chandrasana, 25
Ardha Padma Paschimottanasana, 36; preparation for, 35
Ardha Padmasana, 28, 64, 70; preparation for, 35
Arthritis, 44
Asanas. *See* Postures
Auspicious Pose. *See Swastikasana*
Ayurvedic medicine, 76, 79
Back, 27, 43, 44, 48, 52, 66; injuries, 33, 55; lower, 13, 16, 22, 25, 38, 40, 42, 44, 47, 48, 53, 54, 56, 58; muscles of, 12, 33, 44, 46, 54, 55; pain in, 3, 42, 43, 51; strain, 54, 55; upper, 32. *See also* Spinal discs; Spine Back Stretch Posture. *See Paschimottanasana*
Baddha Konasana, 28, 31, 70
Balance; inner state of, 48, 76; physical, 3, 16, 17, 18, 72
Bellows Breathing. *See Bhastrika*
Bharadvajasana, 44
Bhastrika, 61, 63-64, 73, 76; *Shambhavi*, 63. *See also* Pranayama
Blood, 50, 61
Blood pressure: high, 14, 21, 50, 51, 64; low, 23
Bound Angle Pose. *See Baddha Konasana*
Bow Posture. *See Dhanurasana*
Brain, 61, 63, 76
Breath control, 4, 61. *See also Bhastrika*; Full Yogic Breath; Pranayama

Breathing: during postures, 3, 4; during meditation, 73-74; increasing capacity, 4, 61; shallow, 61; techniques, 61-64. *See also* Breath control
Bridge Pose. *See Setu Bandhasana*
Cardiovascular system, 4
Cat Pose. *See Vidalasana*
Chest, opening of, 19, 21, 25, 40, 42, 44
Chin Mudra, 63, 64, 66
Circulatory system, 4, 12, 29, 43, 50
Concentration, 16, 18, 72
Constipation, 38, 42, 50, 53
Corpse Pose. *See Shavasana*
Counterposes, 12, 53
Cross-Legged Twist, 47
Dandasana, 28
Dhanurasana, 42
Digestive system, 4, 29, 30, 42, 46, 51, 54, 68, 77, 79. *See also* Abdomen; Intestines
Discs. *See* Spinal discs
Diseases, 37, 63, 66, 72-73, 79
Downwards-Facing Dog Pose. *See Adho Mukha Svanasana*
Dynamic Plow Movement, 15
Ear-Pressing Posture. *See Karnipidasana*
Easy Posture. *See Sukhasana*
Elimination, 30, 54
Endocrine system, 4
Eyes, pressure in, 50
Face of a Cow Pose. *See Gomukhasana*
Fatigue, 3, 4, 14, 23, 60, 62
Feet, 70; flat, 29
Female organs, 13, 37
Food, 3, 77, 78, 79; before and after practices, 3, 63, 77
Frog Pose *See Mandukasana*
Full Yogic Breath, 61-62
Gheranda Samhita, 1, 37, 66
Gomukhasana, 32
Halasana, 49, 50, 51

Half-Lotus Backstretching Posture. *See Ardha Padma Paschimottanasana*
Half-Lotus Posture. *See Ardha Padmasana*
Half Moon Pose. *See Ardha Chandrasana*
Hamstring muscles, 3, 4, 12, 14, 23, 26, 28, 33, 58. *See Also* Legs; Thighs
Hatha Yoga, viii, 1-3, 77, 81. *See also* Postures
Hatha Yoga Pradipika, 1, 37
Head on Knee Pose. *See Janushirshasana*
Headstand, 48, 76
Health, 1-3, 66, 77, 79
Heart, 21, 23, 37, 50, 61, 64
Hero Pose. *See Virasana*
Hips, 13, 19, 20, 24, 30, 31, 34, 35, 39, 54, 56, 58. *See also* Joints
Holding Big Toe Pose. *See Padangusthasana*
I Am That, (Swami Muktananda), 74
Inquiry, self, viii
Intense Foot Stretch Pose. *See Prasarita Padottanasana*
Intense Side Stretch Pose. *See Parsvottanasana*
Intense Stretch Pose. *See Uttanasana*
Intestines, 36, 46; gas in, 53, 63; *See also* Abdomen; Digestion; Elimination
Janushirshasana, 34
Jathara Parivartanasana, 53, 56
Joints, 4, 12, 28, 48
Karnipidasana, 52
Knees, 16, 20, 22, 29, 30, 31, 34, 35, 67; pain in, 3, 29, 31, 33, 36, 67, 70
Konasana, 12
Kriyas, 2-3, 73
Kundalini, viii, 2-3, 63, 72-73, 80
Leg-Lifting Posture. *See Uttana Padasana*
Legs, 4, 12, 14, 16, 17, 18, 19, 20, 21, 22, 23, 24, 27, 29. *See also* Hamstring muscles; Knees; Thighs

Locus Pose. *See Shalabhasana*
Lotus Posture. *See Padmasana*
Lungs. *See* Breathing, increasing capacity
Mandukasana, 38
Mantra, 2, 60, 72-74; *Om Namah Shivaya*, 74; *So'ham*, 74
Marichyasana, 45-46
Meditation, viii, 1-3, 16, 47, 60, 61, 63, 66, 67, 71-74, 76, 77, 78, 79; during illness, 76; postures, 65-71; preparation for, 31. *See also* Posture, for meditation
Menstruation, 39; disorders of, 23; practice during, 3, 50
Mind, viii, 4, 18, 23, 33, 48, 61, 63, 66, 68, 72-74, 78
Mountain Pose. *See Tadasana*
Nadis, 2, 66
Neck, 32, 48, 49, 50, 53; pain in, 3, 50
Nervous system, 3, 33, 37, 38, 48, 50, 61, 76. *See also* Spine, nerves of
Obesity, 37, 56
Padangusthasana, 27
Padmasana, 28, 63, 64, 66, 70-71, 73; preparation for, 35
Pain. *See* Back, pain in; Knees, pain in
Parathyroid gland, 48
Parsvakonasana, 20
Parsvottanasana, 24
Paschimottanasana, 37
Pavana Muktasana, 53
Pelvis, 12, 16, 25, 43, 54
Posture, 15, 17, 28; for meditation, 2-3, 28, 34, 48, 66, 72-73. *See also* Shoulders, round
Postures, viii, 1-3, 81; practice during illness, 3, 76; sequence of, 12, 52. *See also*, Hatha Yoga; Meditation, postures; *names of individual postures*; Routines, Hatha Yoga
Prana, 1-3, 16, 61, 63, 66, 72-73, 76, 77

Pranayama, 2, 61, 72-73, 76. *See also Bhastrika*; Full Yogic Breath
Prasarita Padottanasana, 26
Pregnancy, 13, 30, 55, 64
Props, viii
Reclining Toe-Holding Pose. *See Supta Padangusthasana*
Relaxation, 23, 60, 62
Respiratory system, 4, 50
Right Angle Pose. *See Konasana*
Routines, Hatha Yoga, 3, 81
Salutation to the Sun. *See Surya Namaskar.*
Sarvangasana, 48, 49, 51, 76; Modified, 50
Sciatica, 25, 32, 33, 58, 68
Seated Angle Pose. *See Upavistha Konasana*
Self, inner, viii, 3, 12, 72-74, 78
Setu Bandhasana, 48, 53
Sex, 78
Shakti, 3, 72-73, 76, 77
Shaktipat, viii, 2, 76
Shalabhasana, 40-41, 42
Shavasana, 4, 60, 62, 63, 73
Shiva Samhita, 37
Shiva Sutras, 66
Shoulders, 12, 21, 32, 44, 48, 50; joints of, 14; round, 24. *See also* Posture
Siddha Guru, viii, 2, 73, 76
Siddhasana, 63, 66, 73
Siddha Yoga, 2, 76
Side Angle Pose. *See Parsvakonasana*
Sleep, 50, 77
Spinal Discs, 4, 17, 33, 40, 44. *See also* Back; Spine
Spine, viii, 4, 12, 14, 15, 16, 17, 33, 40, 42, 43, 44, 47, 50, 52, 63, 67, 73; injury of, 40; nerves of, 12, 33, 40, 44, 46; vertebrae of, 17, 40, 46. *See also* Back; Spinal discs
Squatting, 30
Stick Pose. *See Dandasana*

Stomach-Turning Posture. *See Jathara Parivartanasana*
Sukhasana, 28, 63, 64, 66, 67, 73
Supta Padangusthasana, 53, 57-58
Surya Namaskar, 4-10; 82-83
Swastikasana, 28, 64, 69
Tadasana, 17
Teacher, need for, 2, 42, 43, 50, 51, 64, 73
Tension, 3, 4, 48, 50, 61, 72
Thighs, 26, 39, 40
Thunderbolt Pose. *See Vajrasana*
Thyroid gland, 48
Tree Pose. *See Vrikshasana*
Triangle Pose. *See Trikonasana*
Trikonasana, 19
Upavistha Konasana, 38-39
Upward-Facing Dog Pose. *See Urdhva Mukha Svanasana*
Urdhva Mukha Svanasana, 8, 43
Uttana Padasana, 54, 55
Uttanasana, 23
Varicose veins, 29, 50
Vajrasana, 64, 68
Vidalasana, 13
Virabhadrasana, 21, 22
Virasana, 28, 29
Vital Organs, 50
Vrikshasana, 18
Warrior Pose. *See Virabhadrasana*
Whole Body Posture. *See Sarvangasana*
Wind-Releasing Posture. *See Pavana Muktasana*
Yoga Sutras (Patanjali), 66, 67, 72-73
Yogic movements. *See Kriyas*

SYDA Publications

Books by Swami Muktananda

I Have Become Alive   Secrets of the inner journey
Play of Consciousness   Muktananda's spiritual autobiography
Satsang with Baba   (Five Volumes) Questions and answers
Where Are You Going?   A guide to the spiritual journey
The Perfect Relationship   The Guru/disciple relationship
Secret of the Siddhas   Swami Muktananda on Siddha Yoga and Kashmir Shaivism
Does Death Really Exist?   A perspective on death and life
Mystery of the Mind   How to deal with the mind
Reflections of the Self   Poems of spiritual life
Muktananda—Selected Essays   Edited by Paul Zweig
Meditate   Muktananda's basic teaching on meditation
In the Company of a Siddha   Muktananda talks with pioneers in science,
    consciousness and spirituality
Light on the Path   Essential aspects of the Siddha path
Mukteshwari I & II   Poetic aphorisms
I Am That   The science of Hamsa mantra
Kundalini: The Secret of Life   Muktananda's teachings on our innate
    spiritual energy
Getting Rid of What You Haven't Got   Informal interviews and talks
Small books of aphorisms: *I Welcome You All With Love, God is With You,
    A Book for the Mind, I Love You*, To Know the Knower and *The Self
    Is Already Attained*

Books about Swami Muktananda

The Glory of the Guru   A photo essay of Swami Muktananda with his words
    on the Guru

Other Books

Nectar of Chanting   Sacred chants sung regularly in Siddha Meditation Ashrams
Lalleshwari   Poems of a great woman saint
Hatha Yoga for Meditators   A detailed guide to Hatha Yoga
Shree Guru Gita   Word-by-word translation with transliteration and
    Sanskrit script

Monthly Publications

Siddha Path   Magazine of SYDA Foundation

Also available in Braille

*For more information about these books as well as foreign translations, write
SYDA Bookstore, PO Box 600, South Fallsburg, NY 12779*

Siddha Meditation is practiced in more than 400 Ashrams and Centers around the world. For information regarding the one nearest you, contact:

Gurudev Siddha Peeth
PO Ganeshpuri (PIN 401206)
District Thana, Maharashtra
India

SYDA Foundation Centers Office
P.O. Box 600,
South Fallsburg, NY 12779
(914) 434-2000